Praise for Dr. Alexander Loyd and
The Healing Code

"You almost have to have a process like The Healing Code to change the wrong beliefs that are keeping you from the life and health you want."

—Bruce Lipton, PhD, former cell biology
researcher at Stanford and author of the
bestselling *Biology of Belief*

"I have found no other process that is as elegantly simple, effortlessly learnable, inherently portable, profoundly effective, and fundamentally timeless. The highest commendation I can give is that I use it for myself, my family, and my patients."

—Merrill Ken Galera, MD, medical director of
The Galera Center, former lead physician
of Dr. Mercola's Natural Health Center

"For many years I was a writer for *Alternative Medicine Magazine*, among others. I have *seen it all* when it comes to natural health. The Healing Codes are the easiest and most effective 'do-it-yourself' healing techniques I have ever found! They work consistently, predictably, and quickly on a wide range of issues. In other words, '*it's the real deal*'!"

—Dr. Christopher Hegarty, bestselling author
and consultant to more than 400 *Fortune*
500 companies

THE HEALING CODE

THE HEALING CODE

6 Minutes to Heal the Source
of Your Health, Success,
or Relationship Issue

Alex Loyd, PhD, ND with
Ben Johnson, MD, DO, NMD

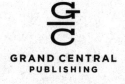

GRAND CENTRAL
PUBLISHING

NEW YORK   BOSTON

Copyright 2010 by Alexander Loyd

Hachette Book Group supports the right to free expression and the value of copyright. The purpose of copyright is to encourage writers and artists to produce the creative works that enrich our culture.

The scanning, uploading, and distribution of this book without permission is a theft of the author's intellectual property. If you would like permission to use material from the book (other than for review purposes), please contact permissions@hbgusa.com. Thank you for your support of the author's rights.

Grand Central Publishing
Hachette Book Group
1290 Avenue of the Americas, New York, NY 10104
grandcentralpublishing.com
twitter.com/grandcentralpub

First Grand Central Life & Style trade paperback edition: September 2013
First Grand Central Publishing trade paperback edition: October 2019

Grand Central Publishing is a division of Hachette Book Group, Inc. The Grand Central Publishing name and logo is a trademark of Hachette Book Group, Inc.

The publisher is not responsible for websites (or their content) that are not owned by the publisher.

ISBNs: 978-1-4555-0200-4 (trade paperback), 978-1-4555-0446-6 (ebook)

Printed in the United States of America

LSC-C

20 19 18 17 16 15 14 13 12

This book is dedicated to YOU, my reader.
My hope and prayer is that this will be the end of
your search or the beginning of the solution, as it was
for my wife, Hope (Tracey), me, and so many others.
May God guide and guard your heart, as he did ours.

—Dr. Alexander Loyd

CONTENTS

PART TWO
Solutions to Healing Virtually Any Health, Relationship or Success Issue

ACKNOWLEDGMENTS

This book would never have happened without a number of people, for whom I am most grateful.

Ben Johnson, thanks for joining me as a friend and brother in this mission. To Tom and Mary Ann Costello, thanks for your marvelous spirit and having my back for the last seven years. To Ken Johnston, for your steady hand of integrity on the wheel. To Lorrie Rivers for helping me get started on this, and all the laughter. To Judith White for handling the details with such love and grace over all the years. To Diane Eble, for helping me get it finished—and so much more.

To my mentor, Larry Napier, thank you for your love and putting me on the heart path.

Many thanks also to my wife, Hope (Tracey), and my boys for putting up with all the note taking at weird times. To God, for something to write about—I am yours!

Everything in this book that is good and true has been a gift from God. I give him the honor and credit, and offer it to you with great joy. Anything in these pages that is not good and true, is all mine, and I ask your forbearance and forgiveness in advance. This book, like The Healing Codes® company, is a calling, not a business. We are on a mission to turn the focus of the world to the issues of the heart, one person at a time. This is the source of your problems, and the solution. This calling started with the love of my life, my wife of twenty-three years—Hope. It continues with my sons, Harry and George, who have taught me much more about love and truth than I will ever teach them. I love YOU forever!

—Alexander Loyd

I want to acknowledge Dr. Alex Loyd for his perseverance in getting this life-changing knowledge out to hurting people with life issues (all of us). The incubation period has been long and the delivery process difficult, but to overcome and triumph is a glorious thing. This book is about changing your life on a primary level—not by working harder or striving more fervently but through understanding and applying simple physics to the body to allow it to heal itself. The body is the healer endowed from above with that ability. The Healing Code is the tool that unchains the healer so that it can do its work. Profoundly simple—most great discoveries are. Alex, I'm deeply grateful to you for the discovery that saved my life.

—Ben Johnson

FOREWORD

Jordan Rubin

The Healing Code developed by Dr. Alex Loyd is a revelation to all who are desperately searching for answers to the challenges they face in their everyday lives.

During my two-year battle with several incurable illnesses, I visited seventy experts in conventional and alternative health, desperate for a cure. After conquering my own diseases through active faith in God and following natural health principals, I went on a mission to transform the health of this nation and world one life at a time. In my quest to find the most effective foundational keys to unlock the health potential of the body, soul and spirit, I have evaluated hundreds of healing modalities, most with mixed results at best.

I was introduced to The Healing Codes by a friend, and I have to admit that at first I was a bit skeptical. Once I heard and read the amazing testimonials of changed lives, and found out that The Healing Codes system was discovered after twelve years of prayer, is completely in harmony with the Bible, and is steeped in science, I wanted to learn more. Shortly thereafter I had the opportunity to spend time with Dr. Alex Loyd. If I had any doubts, they were erased: Alex is a walking testimony to the system he developed.

Not only has Alex facilitated his own family's physical and emotional health breakthroughs, his compassion for those in need and willingness to help people at all costs make him unlike anyone I have ever known. Alex is one of the most contented, giving and peaceful men I have ever met. I have watched Alex Loyd and The Healing Codes dramatically improve the health of friends and family, producing measurable results physically, spiritually, mentally and emotionally.

Yet it wasn't until I was dealing with a great personal crisis that I realized the true power that lies in The Healing Codes. When facing what seemed like insurmountable odds, I worked with Alex daily for a period of forty days and diligently used The Healing Codes to resolve and heal the issues of my heart, many of which I didn't know existed. During this process I was able to almost effortlessly remove painful past experiences and truly forgive those who had hurt me over the years and, more importantly, seek forgiveness on behalf of those I had hurt. I experienced yet another God-given miracle in my life in body, soul and spirit, and I owe much gratitude to Dr. Alex Loyd and The Healing Codes.

This book is based on that system and gives you the essence of what makes it work. With *The Healing Code* you have so much more than just a book. Right now you hold in your hands the keys to unlock your own God-given health potential.

If you utilize the tools in *The Healing Code*, you can achieve true forgiveness, banish wrong beliefs and heal the issues of your heart that are causing stress, failure and even physical disease in your life. Yet as powerful as The Healing Code principles are, they won't work by themselves. You must diligently practice the Healing Code techniques and use the tools, such as the Heart Issues Finder. I urge you to take the time to develop your personalized Healing Code program using the tools in Chapters Eleven and Twelve, you'll be amazed at the quick and effective "Instant Impact" technique that takes 10 seconds to eliminate stress, negative emotions, and increase energy for the day. But it won't do you any good unless you use it when you need it!

Today in America, we hear a great deal about health REFORM. If you utilize the powerful tools available to you in *The Healing Code*, you will see your health and life TRANSFORM from the inside out.

I have benefited greatly from the revelation and wisdom I've received from Dr. Alex Loyd. Now it's time for you to begin your own journey to extraordinary health with *The Healing Code*.

Jordan S. Rubin, NMD, PhD

New York Times bestselling author of more than 20 health and wellness books

Host of the *Extraordinary Health* television program

Founder and CEO, Garden of Life

THE HEALING CODE

PREFACE

The Discovery that
Changed Everything

What do you want most in life? Loving relationships? Having a health issue resolved? Peace? Achievement in an area where you have always felt more capable than your results indicate? Fulfillment that could be measured in a thousand different ways? How can you attain whatever the "thing" is that keeps you awake at night or that quickens your heartbeat?

What I (Alex)[1] want to share with you is a way to attain these things in your life, a way that was given to me in 2001 as a gift of God.

You see, back in 2001, I was the one wanting all these things. The story of the previous twelve years of my life had been sadness, depression, frustration, blocked goals, and helplessness—helplessness in a situation that brought pain and agony to not only myself but my family for those twelve long years. Every time it looked like things were going to improve a little bit, they would slide right back into the despair that had characterized our life together.

What was this problem? Tracey and I said "I do" in 1986 believing that our life would be a "happily ever after" story. Within six months Tracey was crying at the drop of a hat,

---

1 Unless otherwise indicated, when the first person is used, it refers to Alex Loyd.

binging on chocolate chip cookies, and frequently hiding in the bedroom with the door locked. In spite of the fact that living with me could probably do that to anyone on planet Earth, I was very concerned. None of this had happened to her before, and Tracey didn't seem to know why she was so sad, besides being married to me, of course. We soon found out that Tracey was clinically depressed and probably had been for most of her life. In fact, depression and anxiety ran through her family like a commercial lawn mower through foot high grass. Several members of her family have committed suicide in the last thirty or so years.

DESPERATE FOR HELP

We tried everything: counseling, therapy, vitamins, minerals, herbs, prayer, alternative emotional release techniques ... everything! Tracey read a library of psychology, self-help, and spiritual books over these years. I don't know how much money we spent in those twelve years of searching—the last time we totaled it up it was in the tens of thousands of dollars. Some of the things we tried are wonderful practices that we still follow, and a few of them helped, but Tracey was always still depressed.

We thought antidepressants would be the answer. I can vividly remember being awakened in the middle of the night by Tracey's screaming. Turning on the light, I was horrified to see that Tracey was sitting in blood. It was on her, on her gown, and on the sheets all around her. She was screaming and weeping at the same time. I reached for the phone to call 911, thinking that Tracey was hemorrhaging internally. I wondered if she would make it, and how I would raise our six-year-old son if she didn't. It was at about that thought that I realized what had happened–Tracey had been clawing her legs with her fingernails while asleep until she eventually clawed so much skin off of her legs that they bled out onto the sheets. There were many more side effects of the antidepressants, but this one was the worst.

The symptoms of the depression itself were far worse. Once Tracey took a depression self-test that was in the back of a book she was reading and scored in the severely depressed range. I started looking through the test to see how she had answered questions and was shocked to see that she had answered "yes" to a question that asked if she thought about wanting to die most days. She told me that she was too chicken to ever act on it, but that she frequently thought how nice it would be to just veer off the road into a concrete embankment and have the pain all be over.

The depression negatively affected every aspect of our life and family. Many times we were stressed to the breaking point. After being married for three years, Tracey and I both wanted out. The only thing that stopped us was the belief that God had something better in mind. Tracey and I had a recommitment service and renewed our vows–we were truly in it "for better or worse."

The one thing I never lost was hope, and it was that hope that kept me struggling and searching for ways to help Tracey. I searched my way through two doctoral programs, through countless seminars and workshops, through dozens and dozens of books on how to fix the problem. None of these yielded the answers that I was looking for. Lessons learned? Absolutely. Greater maturity? You bet. A belief that I would find the answer? Always.

And then it happened. It happened over a three-hour period. It was like I was the only person on planet Earth, although there were people all around me....

THE BLUEPRINT FOR HEALING

I had been in Los Angeles for a seminar on alternative methods of psychology and was in the airport waiting to board my plane home. My cell phone rang, and when I picked it up I heard the word "Hi." As soon as I heard it, chills ran all over my body. Tracey was severely depressed. She was weeping and said that our son, Harry (who was six), did not understand her being sick in this kind of way. If I had been home I could have knocked out her symptoms with some techniques I knew. However, I was powerless to help her from three thousand miles away. I talked and prayed with her until the stewardess made me turn my phone off. I then started doing what I had done every single day for the previous twelve years–I prayed for Tracey.

What happened next is the reason I am writing this book. The best way I can put it is: God downloaded into my mind and heart what we now call *The Healing Codes*®.

Don't misunderstand me ... there were no angels outside the window of the 737. There was no fog or mist rolling down the fuselage. I heard no heavenly music playing. But what I experienced was so different from anything I had ever been a part of before that I knew it was an answer to those twelve years of daily prayer. I saw the answer in my mind's eye like I have many, many other ideas before–yet it was not the same. You know what I'm talking about if you have ever thought of something and said, "What a great idea!" Well, that's what this was like, only it was like having *someone else's* great idea deposited into my head. It was like I was watching it on TV. It was in my mind but it was not of me. I was "reading" a blueprint of a healing system that I had never studied. The revelation was of a physical mechanism in the body that would heal a spiritual issue—wrong beliefs. I was shown a system that explained how to counteract the true source of all life's issues by doing simple exercises that involved using the hands. So ... I wrote it down, and wrote it down, and wrote it down some more. I wrote until my hand was cramping and I literally said out loud (I remember because I looked around embarrassed that someone might have heard me), "God, you're either going to have to slow down or remind me of this; I can't write that fast!"

When I got home, following this God-given blueprint eliminated the problem that had dominated my life for more than a decade. In 45 minutes, my wife's clinical depression was gone. As I write this it's now more than eight years later, and Tracey has never taken another medication and feels great every day. Yes, Tracey's depression came back after that initial 45 minutes, but within three weeks of doing "The Healing Codes" daily her depression was gone for good. After the years we had been through, painfully searching for something—anything—that would bring normality and peace to our life, I don't know the words to describe the joy and exhilaration this brought to me, my wife and my sons (we now have two). In fact, in 2006 Tracey legally changed her name to Hope. After all the depressed years when she felt hopeless, she no longer felt like the same person. She was now Hope.

After that fateful night when I discovered what we later named The Healing Codes, I was just as excited the following Monday morning when I went to my private practice with plans to integrate this new protocol into working with dozens of people who could have described their lives in words similar to mine. Many pains, many frustrations, many heartaches, many people searching for answers. As I started sharing The Healing Codes with my clients, what happened was exactly what I thought would happen: depression was healed; anxiety was replaced by peace; relationship problems melted away. And even more serious mental and emotional problems seemed to heal consistently, predictably and even quickly in most cases.

THE CIRCLE OF HEALING WIDENS

What I had not expected is what happened six weeks later. A precious client of mine asked if she could speak privately with me for a few moments. She had a puzzling look on her face that I'd never seen before, and stated to me that she could not recall having told me that she had multiple sclerosis (MS). I'm sad to say that I immediately flashed back to one of my doctoral psychology classes on ethics and legal issues and the concern crossed my mind that this was a lawsuit waiting to happen. I rather embarrassedly and nervously looked through her file, saying to her that I could not recall that but let's take a look, when I realized that that was not at all why she was asking the question.

Now feeling compassion and love, I closed the file, put it away, looked her dead in the eye, and said, "I don't remember that either. Why do you ask?" Well, she burst out weeping, almost uncontrollably. When she calmed down, she explained that she had just come from Vanderbilt Hospital in Nashville, where she had learned that she did not have MS anymore. I was deeply moved by the situation and started crying myself.

Tears then turned to laughter and we started laughing. I asked her: "How did you do that? Please tell me so that if I have another client I can share with them what they can do as well. This is wonderful… I am so happy for you."

Then it came: She stated that it was The Healing Codes I'd had her doing for the last six weeks that were responsible for the healing. It had to be—it was the only thing different that she had done.

Well, I thought this was an anomaly. An exception. A one-time unusual response. Until a couple of weeks later I heard a similar story concerning cancer. And then not long after that, diabetes. And then migraine headaches. The early stages of Parkinson's disease. And on, and on, and on.

It was at this point that I knew that what I'd received at 30,000 feet that day was much, much more than I'd hoped or prayed for. I realized the wonderful health ramifications it could have on the world, but I knew no one would believe just because I said it. In fact, most people wouldn't even believe these wonderful stories of healing at all. They sounded too incredible … too fantastic … too sensational. We are bombarded every day with the "sensational" that turns out to be disappointing when applied to our own lives and circumstances.

THE SEARCH FOR VALIDATION

In order for me to bring this to the world, I needed to be convinced in my own mind and heart of two things. One was that it was in harmony with my own spiritual beliefs. For two or three weeks I "hit the pause button" and took time to pray, talk to my minister and to my spiritual mentor, and search Scripture to understand whether this was in harmony with the Bible. At the end of that period, I was convinced that this method of healing is actually more in harmony with the Bible than anything offered either by traditional or alternative medicines. It heals exactly what the Bible emphasizes, and does so according to the way God created the universe and our bodies.[2]

The second thing I had to be convinced of was that The Healing Codes could be validated, scientifically and medically. I had to do this because I was beginning to realize that if this was as good as I thought, I would need to make some radical changes in my life to tell the world about it. I would have to essentially walk away from my private practice. You have to understand, I had worked for five years for my doctorate degree, and those years were a struggle. Not only did we have Tracy's depression to contend with, but I was working two side jobs, going to graduate school full time, paying tuition and supporting a growing family (my first son was born during that time). There were many times when we ate peanut butter or rice and beans for dinner. When I got my degree, within a year I had a six-month waiting list for clients. My private practice as a therapist was thriving, and we were finally enjoying the fruit of our labor.

As wonderful as the healing was that I saw in Tracey and my clients from The Healing Codes, I had to be convinced in my own mind that it was really as good as it seemed. I needed proof.

For the next year and a half I set out to prove to myself that this really was better than anything else out there. I turned to the Heart Rate Variability (HRV) test, the gold standard

---

2 If you would like to know more specifically how I came to this conclusion, there is information on the website you will have access to when you register the book at www.thehealingcodebook.com. Look for "Spiritual Underpinnings."

medical test for measuring stress in the autonomic nervous system. I'd done enough research to know that just about every problem you can imagine has at some time, in some form, in some way, been traced back to stress. I believed that—if The Healing Codes really healed almost anything and everything in the way they seemed to—they had to be removing stress from the body, because in most cases the physical issues that had been healed were not the ones being directly addressed. In fact, the only issues ever addressed by The Healing Codes, past, present, and future, are spiritual issues of the heart.

AMAZING RESULTS

The results of the year and a half of testing with Heart Rate Variability were way beyond what I had hoped for. A medical doctor told me that the results I received had never happened before in the history of medicine. What were these results? Simply that the majority of the time, The Healing Codes remove enough stress from an out-of-balance autonomic nervous system to allow it to come back into balance in 20 minutes or less, and most people (77 percent) are still in balance 24 hours later when tested again. According to available literature going back thirty years, as researched by Dr. Roger Callahan in his recent book *Stopping the Nightmares of Trauma*, the least amount of time it has taken for any therapy to remove this much stress from the body was six weeks. In essence, if you connect the dots, The Healing Codes seem to be removing from the body, in 20 minutes or less, the one thing that is the source of almost all our problems.

While my own test results were not a clinical or double blind study, they were all I needed to show open-minded people that there is hope for their problem. I knew that I had found what I had been looking for, what many people thought was impossible: something that healed the source, not just symptoms—and something that lasted. I had what I needed to be able to walk away from my private practice and start The Healing Codes organization from my basement, with no advertising and very little money. I felt I now had a responsibility to help other people who were hurting as Tracey and I were for twelve years. I am thrilled beyond words to offer you this gift that was given to me by God back in May, 2001 so that you can heal your life as many people around the world have healed theirs.

I (Ben) concur with this. In fact, one of the reasons I came on board to help bring The Healing Codes wider exposure is the remarkable results I experienced, and subsequently saw my patients experience from using this mechanism. Here's what happened to me.

BEN'S STORY

In 1996 it could be said that I was "living the good life" in Colorado Springs, Colorado. My medical practice was exceptional, the patients were wonderful, and my side business of real estate had been very successful. I was enjoying my family and had plenty of time for hunting, fishing and skiing. Life was good!

During this time, my father had undergone triple bypass surgery and then needed his carotid arteries cleaned out because his leg arteries were clogged. He asked me about some unconventional therapies, which were not FDA approved. As he began to recover and his arteries cleared out I became intrigued. The more I looked at herbs and nutritional supplements, as well as off-label uses of FDA approved agents, the more I realized that I had just been treating symptoms, not allowing the disease state to change to wellness.

I began to become disillusioned with drugs and their myriad side effects. There were whole worlds of effective therapies out there that no one had told me about in my formal medical education. I knew I needed to learn more about them. The adventure had begun.

I returned to my native state of Georgia, where I began to devour all the material that I could find on herbs, nutritional supplements, homeopathy, and other alternative medical therapies. It was like going to medical school all over again! I eventually decided there was so much information out there that I needed formal training. I went back and got my Naturopathic Medical Degree (NMD).

Since then, I have strived to offer my patients the best of both worlds. I am combining viable conventional medical approaches with appropriate alternative therapies to create the most effective healing programs for my patients. By doing so, I have achieved much more success working with chronic degenerative diseases, including cancer—an area I eventually chose to specialize in—than I'd previously achieved using conventional medicine alone. Despite my significantly improved success rate, however, like any other physician, I still experienced cases where, no matter what methods I employed, the patient did not respond. It was these cases that kept me searching for a healing method that might work for everyone, regardless of their situation.

DISEASE IS MORE THAN PHYSICAL

One of the great obstacles that I have faced as an integrative cancer physician is the emotional/spiritual issues that my patients have to overcome in order to get well. I have literally had patients die after they became free of their cancer because they could not overcome anger, fear, feeling unloved, unforgiveness, or other issues in their lives. To help my patients more effectively deal with their unresolved emotional/spiritual issues, I investigated and was trained in many therapies, including traditional counseling, Thought Field Therapy (TFT), Emotional Freedom Technique (EFT), Healing Touch, Tapas Acupressure Technique (TAT), Quantum Techniques, and others.[3] Some of these helped to an extent, and some helped more than others. But none was adequate to the task of being able to work for everybody.

The truth of the matter is that we seldom run across a truly new therapy, especially one that can potentially change the landscape of medicine as we know it. Just think of the possibilities of a world without Prozac, Lipitor, insulin, or anti-hypertensives. When this coincides with our own personal point of need it can be a truly phenomenal event. I didn't know it at the time, but the new therapy I was searching for is The Healing Codes,[4] developed by Dr. Alex Loyd, whom I am pleased today to call my friend and partner.

In my cancer clinic in Atlanta we are very progressive. We look at the many causes of cancer and try to design specific therapies for each one. I believe the causes of cancer are a combination of heavy metals, viruses, cellular oxygen deprivation, metabolic acidosis, and emotional/spiritual

---

3 A number of these modalities have a spiritual world view attached to them. Neither I nor Alex ever ascribed to any of that, but used the modalities that could be scientifically validated, solely for their physical benefits.

4 The Healing Code in this book is based on The Healing Codes® system discovered by Alex Loyd in 2001. Hence the references to the plural. It is all the same system. The Universal Healing Code in this book is the result of these subsequent years of testing with clients from 50 states and 90 countries. We have found that it is the Code that works for just about everyone and everything.

issues. We can deal with heavy metals quite effectively using a variety of intravenous and oral agents. A virus and other viral-like particles are much more difficult to deal with, but they can be handled with certain antiviral preparations and other non-FDA approved agents. Addressing cellular oxygen deprivation (for which Otto Warburg won the Nobel Prize for medicine in 1932 when he proved that lack of oxygen is an important cause of cancer) is a slower process. There are intravenous agents to shift the oxygen hemoglobin disassociation curve. This is intimately related to metabolic acidosis and to ongoing diet changes, which are absolutely necessary. Though not easy, addressing all of these issues remains imminently doable. It was the emotional/spiritual issues that remained a major obstacle to getting my patients well. Finding a solution to that problem became an increasingly important quest for me as I continued my medical practice.

MY DEADLY DIAGNOSIS

During my search for the sake of my patients, I began to have some physical problems of my own, primarily fatigue and muscle fasciculation (involuntary contraction or twitching of muscle fibers). Initially, I tried to ignore them, passing them off as a result of the spinal cord injury that I sustained in 1996. But over time, my condition worsened. Muscles would be jiggling in the calf of my leg and at the same time muscles would be in spasm in my back or my upper arms. You could sit there and watch these muscles just jumping up and down under my skin. In addition, I became quite fatigued, even from walking up a short flight of stairs, and my voice grew weak. I decided it was time to visit my orthopedic surgeon, who is also a personal friend. After he conducted his examination of me, it was with great reluctance that he informed me that his diagnosis was amyotrophic lateral sclerosis (ALS), commonly known as Lou Gehrig's disease. I was not happy with this diagnosis, so I promptly sought out another physician friend for a second opinion. He, too, made the same diagnosis.

I went home and pored over my medical books. What I discovered was pretty grim. Eighty percent of people with Lou Gehrig's disease die within five years of developing symptoms, and I had been experiencing them for at least a year! According to the statistics surrounding this disease, I had just lived 25 to 50 percent of the remainder of my life. Many of my cancer patients had a better prognosis than this.

Shortly after my diagnosis, I attended a seminar where I heard Dr. Alex Loyd speak about his new work—The Healing Codes. I found it quite intriguing that, as he began to work with his counseling patients and they began to heal emotionally, they also began to heal physically. This was entirely unexpected but proved to be true, as he saw more and more patients heal physically. With my new diagnosis in hand I redoubled my efforts to investigate Dr. Loyd's discovery.

SCRUTINIZING THE PHILOSOPHICAL BASIS

The philosophical basis was important to me because if the philosophy was flawed the work would be flawed. As this book will explain in more depth, one of the basic concepts of The Healing Codes method is that all memory is stored as pictures, and some of these pictures have non-truths or lies in them which, if left uncorrected, eventually result in emotional and/or physical disease. I didn't have any problem with memory being stored as pictures, as the brain works quite similarly to a supercomputer. The idea of non-truths or lies in these pictures was a little new to me but it made perfect sense. Everyone back to Freud and beyond had proposed that we tied up energy in an earlier state and were subsequently unable to deal with life's problems later on. What was new was the concept that these events, these pictures, were not true. For instance, if someone felt unloved, was he or she truly unworthy of love? Of course not! If we felt incompetent, did it mean our body and mind were truly incapable of performing that action? Probably not. More likely, we just didn't think we could. So I was okay with that concept of believing non-truths. But how could this translate into disease?

I tried to compare this to a computer model that I could understand. We are created with certain programs. One of our programs is the "self-healing" program. As we believe non-truths, the files of this program become corrupted, causing the program to run more and more slowly and eventually fail. If you could figure out a way to uncorrupt the files … Voila! The body's innate ability to heal itself as designed by God would be restored! This was logical in a computer model and viable in a human model.

But how do you go about removing incorrect data and replacing it with corrected data? This came down to a matter of physics for me, since everything, including digital information, ultimately exists as its most common denominator: energy, with a corresponding vibrational frequency. Any frequency can be changed if we only know how to do so.

TAKING THE PLUNGE

I now felt comfortable with the science and philosophy of The Healing Codes. It was time to take the plunge, so I signed up for an instructional seminar. The instruction was good, and I began to learn some simple techniques used by The Healing

Codes coaches. I also decided to purchase an hour of healing work from Dr. Loyd for my own personal use.

I had two things I wanted to work on immediately. First and foremost was my new diagnosis of Lou Gehrig's disease. I also had a long-standing problem with insomnia, which was so severe that for the last few decades I had not been to sleep without a sleep aid at night. I received a Code for my insomnia to be performed three times each day. The first night, after doing only one Code, I went to sleep and slept all night. For the next five weeks, I did not take a single sleep aid. I'm not going to say that I have never taken one subsequently, as I travel extensively and strange beds and unique noises make for difficult circumstances at times. Nevertheless, my sleep pattern has remained remarkably improved, and I seldom take a sleep aid.

As for my muscle fasciculations, fatigue, and other Lou Gehrig's symptoms—they are gone. After only three months of practicing The Healing Codes, I returned to the surgeon who first diagnosed me. He ran the test for Lou Gehrig's (EMG) and found it to be 100 percent gone. I have been symptom-free since March 2004. For those of you who don't know—there is no cure for Lou Gehrig's disease.

After personally experiencing the results of The Healing Codes techniques, I elected to learn the work in its entirety. I have also trained the staff in my cancer clinic in Atlanta, so that my patients can have the benefits of this great work as well. Based on the results my staff and I are seeing, I now know that I have found the healing method I was searching for. I know of nothing else that addresses and heals emotional and physical issues so effectively and completely.

I recently found myself one Friday night with nothing to do, so my children and I decided to watch a movie. Rather than go out into the cold to the video store, the children combed through our collection. Finding a copy of *2001: A Space Odyssey*, they wanted to know what it was about, having never seen it. As I thought about the movie's theme—that humanity is on the verge of another evolutionary leap—I thought about the rate at which our knowledge in all fields is increasing in an exponential fashion. The same thing is happening in medicine. I have long believed that we are ready to move to a different level in the healing paradigm.

In Chapter Two, a brief history of medicine and healing, you will see clearly why I believe The Healing Codes has made a bold leap into the next step in the healing paradigm. It has avoided the mysticism that usually surrounds such therapies. It is philosophically and scientifically sound. Not to mention that it works! I'm living proof of that!

One last word about The Healing Code being scientifically sound, before we move on. No matter how conclusive testing seems to be, there will always be critics. Typically, they will cite a potential problem common to all testing: The results could be due to the placebo effect (it's all in your head). So if a conservative scientist wants to say "This has not been proven," they can. I had a good friend in the natural health field who had this happen with a wonderful product that had been validated by independent testing from 16 universities. As you might guess, his competitors did not appreciate his success. Quite often, when you get to the bottom of who is throwing the rocks, they have an agenda—it's often not about the studies at all. One of the most wonderful and unexpected things to come out of our year and a half of testing was a wonderful "cherry on top" that answers this potential criticism. Consistently, the fastest and most dramatic healing occurred in animals and infants. The point: IT'S IMPOSSIBLE TO PLACEBO AN ANIMAL OR INFANT! There was absolutely no way that the results we were seeing were from the placebo effect. It had to be real, true source healing. We so greatly appreciate the brave, openminded, world-class scientists and doctors who have supported and endorsed The Healing Code. They have endured criticism from peers for that, but they have been willing to courageously go where the research and results point, even if it is out of the traditional, scientific box. BRAVO!

FOUNDATIONS

(Do Not Skip This!)

There's a saying in the news business to never, never bury the lead.

This chapter is the lead. If you get this, you get everything. So, get this ...

The Three "One Things"

Crazy title, huh? Let us try to explain.

In the original *City Slickers* movie with Billy Crystal, Curly, played by Jack Palance, was the tough, stodgy old cowboy who almost never spoke. But under that rough exterior, Billy Crystal found the wisdom of the ages. In an improbable heart-to-heart between the two, Curly shared with Billy the Secret of Life. The Secret of Life, he said, was one thing. When pressed to name it, Curly refused to divulge what that one thing was. He said Billy would have to find that one thing for himself. And, indeed, everyone needs to find that one thing for themselves.

You see, "One Thing" can make all the difference. Have you ever spoken to someone about their life when suddenly there was a dramatic positive change in their manner? At some point, a sparkle came into their eye as they spoke of one person, one moment, one event, one open door, one breakthrough ... ONE THING.

We want to offer you, right now, three "One Things." We believe that as far as your life, your health, and your prosperity are concerned, these three things make all the difference. Not only are we going to tell you what they are, we're going to prove them to you and share with you a new discovery that can become the sparkle in your eye that you look back on for the rest of your life.

If you do not agree that we have done what we just said we were going to do, then please ask us to return the money you spent for this book.

THE THREE ONE THINGS

One Thing #1: *There is one thing on planet Earth that can heal just about any problem in your life.*

One Thing #2: *There is one thing on planet Earth that will turn off One Thing #1.*

One Thing #3: *There is one thing on planet Earth that will turn One Thing #1 back on.*

ONE THING #1

There is one thing on planet Earth that can heal just about any problem in your life.

What is it? The immune and healing systems of the body.

Think about or write down the top two or three problems in your life. Health problems, career, relationship, finances—it doesn't matter what it is. I'm assuming that unless the problem just arose this very minute, you have already tried something (or many somethings) to resolve or lessen this as a problem in your life. If you haven't, cool! You can start now with the one that will actually fix it. No problem. If you have tried other things, then we believe you're at the end of your search. Here's why. Imagine for a minute that whatever your problem is, you could have God himself reach down and hand you a supernatural pill, liquid, secret, treasure map … in other words, a solution not of this world, guaranteed to work. Boy, would that be awesome! Guess what? You already have it!

Every person has an absolutely miraculous healing system in his or her body that can heal any physical or non-physical issue that a person might have. It's called your immune system. We are born with a self-healing program inside that is designed to be capable of fixing any problem before it becomes a problem. Even if a problem does develop, that's okay, too. The program can fix it once the problem arises.

Awhile back my computer was not working properly. Not being a computer person, I became frustrated by trying everything I knew how to do. Finally, I called a good friend of mine who is a computer whiz kid. After asking a few simple questions, he confidently told me that I needed to defrag my hard drive. I had never heard of such a thing, but was thrilled to discover that it was a simple matter of pushing a couple of buttons. After doing this, my computer ran almost like new. I was amazed that such a wonderful function could be inside my computer and I did not even know it.

Just like the computer's "defrag" program, your immune system is capable of healing any issue you may have with amazing speed and efficiency. I (Ben) can tell you that if you were to ask one important question of just about any doctor or health care practitioner in the world, and they answered honestly, every one of them would answer "no." So what's the question? "Is there any disease or illness that an optimally functioning immune system cannot heal?" Answer: No. In fact, many experts believe (and I concur) that the only healing that ever happens for any person for any health issue happens because of the immune system.

You may be thinking, "But how can I apply this to relationships, or finances, or career, or other non-physical things that may be a struggle in my life?" As you will see later in the book, specifically in Secret #3 (but don't peek!), new discoveries at several of our finest and most highly regarded medical schools have found that the source of illness and disease is also the source of the other problems in our lives. Furthermore, we believe and will present proof to you that we have actually discovered a part of the body's healing system that people have never known about before. We believe this new healing mechanism and how to turn it on can be the One Thing that creates a breakthrough with the struggles of your life.

If you're a reasonably intelligent person and think about this long enough, you're very likely to come up with this question: "If this healing system really can heal anything and it's already inside me, then why do I have the problems in the first place? Why hasn't it already healed them or prevented them from happening?"

We're glad you asked. Because that takes us to One Thing #2.

ONE THING #2

There is one thing on planet Earth that will turn off One Thing #1.

So what is it? Stress. (But probably not what you think of when you think of stress.)

If the immune and healing systems of the body can heal any problem you have, then the thing that turns those systems off must be the one cause of all illness and disease. It is. According to Stanford University Medical School in research released in 1998 by Dr. Bruce Lipton, a highly renowned and respected cell biologist, stress is the cause of at least 95 percent of illness and disease. Dr. Lipton reports that the remaining 5 percent is genetic and was caused, you guessed it, by stress somewhere in the ancestry of that person. Even the US Federal Government, the Centers for Disease Control (CDC), says on their website that 90 percent of all illness and disease is related to stress. Just about any authoritative source you could name agrees—Harvard, Yale, Vanderbilt, The Mayo Clinic, and the list goes on.

Especially notable is what the Harvard Medical School says on their website. "Too much stress for too long creates what is known as 'chronic stress' which has been linked to heart disease, stroke, and may also influence cancer and chronic respiratory diseases. And illness is just the tip of the iceberg. Stress affects you emotionally, as well, marring the joy you gain from life and loved ones."[5]

In other words, whatever problem you have, somehow or another, it probably came from stress. Thus far, we haven't been quite sure what to do about it, because what works for one problem and one person is ineffective for another problem and another person. The conclusion has been painfully clear for decades. If we are going to find a way to heal illness and

5 "Stress Management: Approaches for Preventing and Reducing Stress," Harvard Health Publications, Harvard Medical School, http://www.health.harvard.edu/special_health_reports/stress_Control.htm.

disease at its source, we have to find a way to consistently and predictably heal stress.

And as the Harvard Medical School report said, illness is just one manifestation of stress. If we want to deal with other issues as well—relationship issues, performance issues that affect success—we need to deal with the source. As we will prove to you, stress is also the source of these kinds of issues as well, as evidenced by the fact that when people heal the source of their stress, their relationships improve, their income goes through the roof, and their satisfaction soars.

It's important to note that the kind of stress we're talking about that creates this illness and disease is not based on circumstances that you wish you could change. It is deep-seated stress that lives inside you and is totally independent of your current circumstances. In fact, changing your current circumstances by eliminating things that seem stressful to you may very well have little effect on this stress that turns off our immune system. In our research, more than 90 percent of people who say they are not stressed before they are tested for stress actually *are* under physiological stress, according to their test results. Many of the medical school research studies spoken of above say this very thing—what stresses one person doesn't stress another. It depends on your "internal" programming.

THE REAL QUESTION TO ASK

This means that the first question you should be asking any time you have a problem that you can't seem to get beyond is, "What stress is keeping my immune system from healing this and how do I fix it?" The problem is that this kind of stress can be almost impossible to find, you may not have a clue it's there, and if you do find it, it is literally protected from being fixed (more about all of this later).

On the other hand, you may not realize how good this news is. Why do I say that? Because it's not your fault. The problem and the solution are not based on effort, and everyone has this kind of stress whether they've been good girls or boys or not. So relax and forgive yourself. You don't have to be perfect. We've got what you've been looking for. What do we have? It's ...

ONE THING #3

There's one thing on planet Earth that can turn One Thing #1 back on.

What is it? Healing the issues of the heart!

Let's review real quickly. The human immune and healing systems, when functioning correctly, are designed to heal—and are capable of healing—just about anything. However, a certain kind of stress will turn the immune and healing systems off, or at least turn them down to the point that we develop health or other problems.

The Healing Code can turn the immune and healing systems back on because it heals "issues of the spiritual heart." The Healing Codes® encapsulates the discovery of a system that's been in the body since the dawn of time. How do we know that The Healing Code can turn them on again? Because when we use a gold standard medical test that does not respond even 1 percent to the placebo effect, the results are unprecedented in the history of medicine.

What exactly are these test results? When this Healing Code system in the body is activated, physiological stress disappears, either completely or at least significantly. Using just a little bit of logic, if the one thing on planet Earth that will turn off the immune and healing systems is forced to disappear, then the immune and healing systems should turn back on. That's exactly what we've had the pleasure of watching with people all over the world since the spring of 2001. Not only is The Healing Code mechanism revolutionary, but people tell us that the theory behind The Code had an even bigger impact on their lives. We call the theory "The Seven Secrets."

An amazing aspect of all this is that no Healing Code ever "treats" any health issues. The Healing Codes only address the "issues of the heart" that Solomon wrote about more than 3,000 years ago, when he said in Proverbs 4:23, "Guard your heart above all else, for out of it are all the issues of life." Notice that it says *all* the issues of life come from the heart. This is why scores of people report healing from just about any health issue you can imagine after using The Healing Code.

BEFORE WE GO ANY FARTHER ...

Perhaps you're curious about what The Healing Code is and want to get right to it. That's fine—just turn to Part Two and you'll get all the details of what a Healing Code is and how to do it. But at some point, we do want you to learn The Seven Secrets in Part One. In order to use The Healing Code most effectively, you need to understand how problems develop and what you can do to heal yourself for the rest of your life by getting at the source of your problems.

The Seven Secrets in Part One are as revolutionary as The Healing Code itself, because this theory doesn't deal with symptoms alone, as just about every other self-help system does. Every other system addresses one or more of five areas: emotions; thoughts; conscious beliefs; actions and behaviors; or the physiology of the body. From our research, as outlined in the following pages, we believe these five things are just symptoms. The Healing Code theory and application address issues at the source, not just the symptoms.

So Part One of this book gives a brief history of health care and The Seven Secrets to Life, Health and Prosperity. We will uncover and explain the theory and research that reveal the source of not only all health problems, but just about any other problem as well. We know that's a tall order, but we're quite willing to prove it to you!

Part Two is all about results. Some people might find it interesting to read a book that lets them know why their lives are messed up, but if that's where it ends, most will feel frustrated about being unable to change the problem. This book will not leave you high and dry. Part Two will give you the information you need to start healing the source of your problems and the thing that may be blocking your hopes and dreams. As a bonus, we will also give you a 10-second exercise for dealing with the circumstantial stress that arises in any given day. So Part Two will give you a way to heal both the stress you're all too aware of, and the unconscious stress that is the true, underlying cause of all your other problems.

You may be tempted to put this book down right now. Why? In the past, you've heard one too many "magic bullet" stories. One too many promises of breakthroughs, life change, miracles, and more. We have, too! However, we must tell the truth, and the discoveries and insights and stories that are in this book were the pot of gold at the end of the rainbow of my life search to find the one healing method that was real and could deliver, and the source of healing Ben's Lou Gehrig's disease (ALS). We can't not share this information!

We don't ask you to accept this as truth right now. We ask you only to keep on going and read the rest of this book before you decide. That's our challenge to you. You have several hours of your life to "lose" ... and potentially decades of well-being to gain.

Now that you know The Three One Things and have some background to work with, we'll move on to the heart of the matter. To get what you want, you need to understand what I call "The Seven Secrets to Life, Health, and Prosperity." By understanding these seven critical issues, you will come to know how your problems develop, where they come from, what they consist of, why they resist healing, and finally, the simple mechanism that can start to unwind the fabric of what you don't want in your life.

Before we go there, though, we want to issue a very serious and heartfelt warning.

The information in this book has the power to cause great healing in your life. The mechanism we call The Healing Code can turn off your stress and get your immune system to work the way God intended. You will see amazing changes in your life as a result.

However, there is a purpose to pain, a spiritual purpose, and if The Healing Code helps you deal with the pain but not with the ultimate source of your pain, we have actually done you a disservice.

You see, the deepest healing every person on earth needs is not physical or emotional, but spiritual, and it involves healing any disruption of a relationship with a loving God. That is something only God can do. That is something that is between you and God.

People have told us over and over again that The Healing Code has helped them get issues healed that prevented them from believing in a loving God. One person said, "It's as if the static of my own issues was removed so that I could finally hear the messages God was telling me about the way he truly is, not the distortions caused by my own heart issues."

It is not the intent of this book to tell you how to believe.[6] But it is our fervent hope and prayer that you will come to know the One who created the human body and energy and all the things that make The Healing Code work the way it does. That is the most important healing that can occur, and while The Healing Code can help the process, as a tool, it can't do that job. The Healing Code is a very wonderful tool. But what you ultimately need to grab hold of is the Hand that wields the tool.

---

6 We ourselves are followers of Jesus. When I (Alex) discovered The Healing Codes system, it was in fact a process for me to make sure that this was something I could use in accordance with my own beliefs, as mentioned in the Preface. For more information on our philosophy and beliefs, see "A Word about Us and Our Philosophy" on p. 289.

PART ONE

The Seven Secrets to Life, Health and Prosperity

CHAPTER ONE

Secret #1:
There Is One Source
of Illness and Disease

In order to see the door we're now ready to walk through, let's take a look at the path that brought us here. Let us tell you in advance that the door we see before us has been predicted by the greatest scientific minds of our time for decades, and in some cases even centuries. So this door that we're ready to walk through is a golden door that science has searched for, and what is on the other side is going to change the world of health forever. To say that this is a paradigm shift is an understatement.

As I (Ben) mentioned earlier, I was healed of Lou Gehrig's disease after using The Healing Codes for less than three months. I was so impressed with this program that I have begun lecturing all over the country about The Healing Codes and how they work. This also led to my being the only MD featured in the popular DVD, *The Secret*. One of the things I lecture about is the Five Eras of Healing, because it gives us important background as to where we have arrived at this point in history and may also explain why The Healing Codes could not have been discovered before now.

THE FIVE ERAS OF HEALING

There are five main eras we'll speak about here. The first era was prayer. Before human beings knew or understood nutrition or any type of medicine, all they could do was pray. This may seem a strange place to begin the history of medicine, but let's think about Man in the beginning. When humankind experienced ill health, all they could do was seek the deities for healing. History is replete with idols, religious practices, and ceremonies for healing. In Greek mythology, Apollo was believed to be the primary source of healing, and he transmitted his powers to his son Asclepius, who not only prevented people from dying, but even raised some from the dead. In northern Peru, healing ceremonies are still performed by women called *curanderos*. The curanderos use prayer and sacred objects, cleanse the patient with holy water, and call on the spirit power to help them discover the cause of the affliction and to cleanse and heal them.

Today, God is still sought as the sole source of healing by many cultures, religions, and individuals. Some people through the years have believed that the power of prayer was in the praying itself, while others have believed the source of the power to be supernatural intervention by a greater power. Recently, many scientific studies have indicated the effectiveness of prayer in the area of healing. Dr. Larry Dossey, MD, has written several books on the power of prayer in healing (*Healing Words: The Power of Prayer in the Practice of Medicine; Miracles of Mind: Exploring Nonlocal Consciousness and Spiritual Healing; Reinventing Medicine: Beyond the Mind-Body to a New Era of Healing*, etc). Studies called "The Mantra Study Project" have been conducted at Duke University (Horrigan, 1999) and found that patients with angina gained the most benefit from receiving prayer. People through the ages have prayed because they believe in a higher power. Another theory is that healing flows from belief in healing itself. Science has also proven that belief itself is a very powerful healer. Medicine has dismissed this and even disparaged it, calling it the "placebo effect." Nevertheless, the effect is very real and not to be discounted.

On a more physical level, it didn't take long to figure out that certain leaves, twigs, roots, or bark were valuable in healing. So we began a long history of herb use. This fell into brief disrepute and decreased usage in Western civilization during the twentieth century. However, it has made a tremendous comeback. You can hardly drive down the street without seeing an herb or nutritional shop. In our recent travels lecturing around the world, we hear people talking about vitamin, mineral, and herbal alternatives everywhere we go. This resurgence has been all the more remarkable because it's not the backwoods uneducated, but the very sophisticated intellectuals who have come to the same conclusions about herbs and supplements that others have known for centuries. China has been using herbs from time immemorial—as long as there has been recorded history.

Western civilization has upped the ante on Chinese medicine by trying to concentrate certain parts of plant foods, which has resulted in a huge vitamin/nutritional industry. Bookshelves are full of the findings of modern miracles from plants. Nutrition shops have hundreds of products that have been extremely beneficial to people with virtually every disease.

However, this is coming to a screeching halt. A new law has been passed called "CODEX," promoted by the World Health

Organization, that will limit concentrations of vitamins, minerals, amino acids and essential oils to levels that would fall short of the healing effects that we've experienced for decades. Anything above this will have to be prescribed by a physician and be purchased at a dramatically higher price. You may think that I'm talking about some future event, but any government that has ratified the WHO agreement is already under that law. Even countries like the U.S. with extremely strong constitutions find themselves under this law because treaty law can override constitutional law. CODEX met in Rome in June of 2005 and affirmed the drug-industry-imposed standards in a Codex guidance document entitled "Vitamin and Mineral Guideline." It has already taken effect in Germany, where you can now only get vitamins in significant doses via prescription from a physician. I predict that many governments will move slowly to regulate this industry so that there will not be an outcry from the public. I believe they will try the "frog in the water" approach. This is particularly disturbing when considered in light of the far greater danger of pharmaceutical drugs—especially in this circumstance, over-the-counter pharmaceutical drugs—that with CODEX in effect would be much easier to obtain than vitamins.

One might wonder why governments would pass a law like this, which makes vitamins, minerals and nutrients illegal over the counter but lets much more toxic pharmaceuticals remain restriction free. The pharmaceutical industry does not profit when someone gets well; they only profit when someone treats symptoms month after month and year after year.

This leads into our next era of medicine, the drug/chemical era. Why do I call them chemicals? Very simply, that's what they are. The way most drugs are developed is to find an herb that has a benefit. They then try to break it down and find out the "active" ingredients. Now, this is still not patentable. And remember, there is no profit without exclusivity. So the next step in the process of making a drug is that we have to alter the "active" ingredient so that it's not natural.

Now we have a chemical. You would think that's not so bad, but understand that the organic systems of the body are designed to deal only with organic materials. So we have a substance, a drug that the body can no longer break down. This is called a toxin. We have a whole industry that is built around manufacturing toxins when we could be using natural organic materials that work much more efficiently with the physiology of the body and all of the natural components that are part of the original organic substance or plant. Example: One of the top-selling drugs in history is called Valium. It is not related to Valerian root. This root is one of the best natural sedatives and anti-anxiety agents. There has never been one case in history of a person being addicted to Valerian root. However, no company can patent the Valerian root. It occurs naturally in nature. The chemical creation of Valium, in order to patent and market a more powerful version of the natural Valerian root, has resulted in the need for Valium addiction clinics all over the world.

To continue our journey, next we'll take a look at surgery. Mankind has dabbled with surgery for centuries. However, it remained very crude until the discovery of anesthesia. Prior to this, physicians could only perform what people could tolerate based on their level of pain or how many people you had to hold them down. Alcohol was occasionally used as a general anesthetic. The purpose and value of surgery was to remove something that was life threatening. For instance, if someone had gangrene of the foot, the surgeon would have the person held down and take a hack saw and cut off the leg. Fire was initially used for cautery. Needless to say, we have come a long way in our surgical techniques. However, now not only is surgery used for life-threatening situations, but some would even say it is used frivolously in cosmetic surgery, a booming industry. While statistics indicate that a significant number of surgeries are performed unnecessarily, surgical trauma medicine has been a great gift to civilization and is responsible for the saving of countless lives.

THE FINAL FRONTIER

Now for what you've been waiting for: the golden door. What the greatest scientific minds of our time, starting with Albert Einstein, have predicted has now been discovered, validated, and made available to the general public. Many other great scientists have spoken to this subject, but we will leave this for the Second Secret later in the book. I will begin with a quote from one of those great minds:

"Future medicine will be based on controlling energy in the body."
– Professor William Tiller, Stanford University

That's right, energy is the final frontier. It is the ultimate form of healing. Medicine has been dabbling in it for some years, and even unwillingly been dragged into it, but irresistibly it has arrived. We haven't always known that sunlight had a healing effect. Madame Curie helped us to enter this era with the discovery of radium and X-rays. She also discovered how damaging energy could be. You will learn more about what "energy" is, and how extremely damaging or healing it can be, in the coming chapters. You will also understand why it is the future of health and healing.

BEYOND THE SYMPTOM COMPLEX

The way almost all health problems are diagnosed and treated today is based on what is called a "symptom complex." The symptom complex is used not only in traditional medicine, but also in alternative health care, and it has been used for hundreds of years.

The way a symptom complex works is much like it sounds. The doctor or health care practitioner, problem solver, counselor, or helper, takes note of all the symptoms that a person has. Once they've identified the symptoms, they then consult a book, a chart, or their experience to determine what is the most likely problem based on that particular set of symptoms. Once they've determined what most likely the problem is—this is called a diagnosis—they then move on to treatment, asking, "What is the best way to treat that problem within the standard of practice?" Treatment is largely determined by the methodology of the practitioner. Traditional medical doctors use surgery, medications—things like that. Alternative health care providers use herbs, minerals and vitamins, not to "treat" disease, but to support optimal health. Counselors and therapists teach and advocate thinking about the problem differently and using behavioral techniques, or simply provide the support of a kind ear.

So the symptom complex basically involves three stages:

1. Presentation of symptoms.
2. Diagnosis based on the presenting of symptoms that comes from experience, schooling, or a book.
3. Actual intervention, therapy or treatment of the problem based on the diagnosis.

There are literally thousands of possibilities for each of these three stages. When you talk about health issues, you have physical health and mental health. Other problems would include relational problems, career problems, and peak performance issues (as in athletics, achievement, speaking, and sales). Each of these issues has different possibilities depending on what the issues are that you're dealing with and the methodology of the practitioner. In other words, this process can become extremely complicated and even controversial, because different experts disagree on what the diagnosis should be, and even more so regarding the intervention, therapy or treatment that is needed.

If you want to get an idea of how frustrating this issue can be, go to the Internet and type any health issue into a search engine. It doesn't matter what it is—pick a disease, pick a mental health issue, pick headaches, whatever you want. You'll probably find a lot of interesting information, but you'll also find a tremendous amount of disagreement, not only about what causes the problem, but especially what to do about it. You may very well come away a little bit disillusioned, realizing how much the experts disagree. So if the experts disagree, how in the world does the person who's not an expert, who's just a person with a problem, ferret out and determine what is the best course of action for them without wasting a tremendous amount of time or money; or in the worst case, possibly losing their life because of trying a solution that is not the right one for them?

Let's talk some more about the expense of time and money. Let's say that you did do that Internet search and found that there were ten different suggestions for how to go about dealing with your problem. Let's say you tried six of them before trying the one that benefited you most. In this case you probably wasted a great amount of money and time on the first five that did not help your problem.

Wouldn't it be wonderful if there were one source of all problems? If there were one source of all problems, you could simply address that one thing that is the source in order to solve whatever your problem was. This would have several advantages. You wouldn't waste so much time and money, because you'd only be working on one thing! If there's one source of all problems then it also has to be the source of your problems, so you could feel confident that if you're healing that one source, then you're improving in all directions. You might even go so far as to say, "If I'm healing the one source, then I know I'm doing what is best for my problem."

You could have peace of mind because you know that you're doing what's best—you're working on the one source. You could have peace of mind because you know you're almost definitely saving a lot of money. You could have peace of mind because you know you're saving a lot of precious time and energy because you can go directly to addressing that one source.

The final reason may be the biggest one of all. That is, if there were one source of all problems, and if you have ten problems, you could relieve all of them at one time, because they all go back to that same one source. If you heal that one source, you could actually be healing all ten of the worst problems that are keeping you from having the life you want to have, having the relationships you want to have, having the peace, the prosperity, and the success you want to have. You could be dealing with all of them at the same time rather than having to do it the old way by treating one of them at a time and going through that symptom complex and using a different intervention for each one of them.

So there would be multiple advantages to having only one source of all health problems.

Well, get ready to celebrate, because the one thing that most people in the health field agree on is that there is one source of almost all health problems. That's our first Secret!

SECRET #1: THE ONE SOURCE OF ILLNESS AND DISEASE

Let's go back to our example of doing a Web search on a health problem. Remember our frustration because the experts disagreed on how to treat the problem? Well, the one thing that just about everyone does agree on is that almost all health issues originate from one problem—STRESS! In fact, over the last 10-15 years this has become so universally accepted that even the United States federal government has come out publicly in agreement.

As we stated earlier, the Centers for Disease Control in Atlanta says that 90 percent of all health issues are related to stress. Dr. Bruce Lipton, on the other hand, in research released in 1998 out of Stanford University Medical School, disagrees with the CDC. Based on his laboratory work, Dr. Lipton believes that over 95 percent of all illness and disease is linked to stress.

The major media regularly covers the topic. *The New York Times* online Health Guide points out that "stress can come from any situation or thought that makes you feel frustrated, angry, or anxious. What is stressful to one person is not necessarily stressful to another."

Back in September 2004, *Newsweek* devoted the cover and major issue of the magazine to "The New Science of Mind & Body." Articles covered "Forgiveness and Health," "Stress and Infertility," "Clues to Heart Disease" and more. We'll get back to the idea of "Forgiveness and Health" later on.

Another prominent news magazine, *Time*, on its cover called high blood pressure "the stealth killer" that was spinning out of control. Stress has been identified as a cause of high blood pressure again and again.

I have pages and pages of research on how stress is the source of illness. One article in *USA Today* from May 30, 2004, called "Manage Stress, Manage Illness," cited sources from Harvard, Arizona State University, University of North Carolina, National Heart, Lung and Blood Institute, Michigan Technological University, the American Medical Association (AMA), Tulane University, Indiana University Cancer Center, and the Department of Health and Human Services. Other studies are from the Mayo Clinic, Vanderbilt University, the Yale Stress Center, Harvard Medical School, the CDC, the Anderson Cancer Center, the National Academy of Sciences, Boston University—the list goes on, and is added to every week as new research comes out.

So what does all this mean? It means that the very first question we should be asking ourselves based on the latest research is this: "What is the stress that's causing this and how can I fix it?"

Before we can answer this question, we need to answer another question, "What exactly is stress in the body?"

THE PHYSIOLOGY OF STRESS

What exactly is stress? Is it getting a bill in the mail? Having an argument with a neighbor? Things not going as we planned at work? Concern about our health? You name it, and yes, it can be stressful. However, there is a critical difference between circumstantial issues that we normally think of as stress and physiological stress that results in illness and disease.

Physiological stress, simply put, is when our nervous system is out of balance. The central nervous system can be described using the analogy of a car. If you continually floor the gas pedal, you'll end up breaking something. Likewise, if you ride the brakes, you will end up breaking something. The car is designed to work properly with the gas and brakes working harmoniously in balance. The same can be said of the central nervous system. This system has two parts, just like the gas and brakes on the car. The gas is similar to the sympathetic nervous system (amping things up), while the parasympathetic nervous system works similarly to the brakes (slowing things down). The state-of-the-art test in mainstream medicine for measuring physiological stress is called "Heart Rate Variability" (HRV), and measures the balance or lack of balance in this system. We'll talk more about this test later.

The larger part of the nervous system is called the autonomic nervous system (ANS). "Autonomic" means "automatic," because we don't have to think about it. It happens automatically. In fact, 99.99 percent of everything going on in the body at any given moment is under the autonomic nervous system's control. We have about five trillion bits of information coming into the brain every second. We are only aware of about ten thousand bits.

For instance, you don't think about the food that you ate for lunch in your small intestine. You don't have to think about moving it on to the next segment of the bowel. You don't have to think about adding amylase to break down starch. Or adding lipase to break down fat. You don't have to think about increasing insulin to handle excess sugar. You are not thinking about your kidneys getting rid of the excess sodium because you added extra salt to your food. You're not thinking about your liver detoxifying the pesticides that were on the vegetables, nor about your immune system fighting the bacteria that came in with the food. We could keep on going, but you get the idea. Almost everything that is happening in your body, including your hair growing, is being done automatically. You don't have to think about it. And isn't that wonderful? There wouldn't be enough hours in the day if you had to consciously think about all those things happening!

IT'S ALL ABOUT BALANCE

There are two parts to the ANS, and again, it's all about balance. There is the parasympathetic nervous system (PNS), which is in charge of growth, healing, and maintenance. It encompasses most of the automatic things we were just talking about.

Then there is the sympathetic nervous system (SNS). It's designed to be used much less frequently, yet it plays a huge role in health and sickness. The SNS is what we call the "fight or flight" system. It is the fire alarm. It is intended to save our lives at any given moment, very much like when you're out on the highway in a car. You use the gas most of the time but the brakes may save your life every time you drive.

When we go into fight or flight, many things happen. Blood flow completely changes. It's no longer going to the stomach to digest food. It's no longer going to the frontal lobes of the brain for creative thought. It's no longer going to the kidneys and liver. The lion's share of the blood is now going to the muscles because your body thinks that it is going to have to fight harder or run faster than whatever is threatening your life. So you don't need to digest that food in the bowel or clear the toxins from the liver, balance the electrolytes in the kidneys, or have creative thought, because if you don't survive the next few minutes, all of that doesn't matter. Again, these things happen automatically.

THE CRUCIAL CELLULAR LEVEL OF STRESS

Although they are designed to save your life, these changes, sustained over time by continual stress, can cause damage to organs, especially and directly affecting the immune system. That's what's going on at an organ level. Let's talk for just a minute about what is happening on a cellular level. I have a good friend who is a PhD in nutrition and a naturopathic physician. She had never understood why many people didn't get well or heal when she gave them the proper nutritionals, vitamins and minerals. Now make no mistake about it, she was giving them the right ones. She's a very good doctor. What she didn't fully understand was the effect of stress on a cellular level.

In the Navy, when a ship is attacked, all maintenance, repair, and normal activities cease. Even crew that are sleeping or eating have to "man the battle stations." When the fire alarm (the SNS) goes off, our cells cease their normal growth, healing and maintenance. Why? The fire alarm is only supposed to go off in an emergency, and all of those activities can wait a few minutes while we run or fight to save our lives. The cells literally close up, like a ship battening down the hatches in a time of attack. Nothing is going in or out. You don't see a tender ship coming up beside a battleship to give it food or to unload the garbage during a battle. In the same way, our cells don't receive nutrition, oxygen, minerals, EFAs, etc., nor do they get rid of waste products and toxins while under stress. Everything stops except what is necessary to survive. This results in an environment inside of the cell that is toxic and doesn't allow for growth and repair. In fact, Dr. Bruce Lipton says that this is exactly how we get genetic illness and disease. On the flip side, the same research at Stanford found that cells that were open and in growth and healing mode are literally impervious to illness and disease. Let me state that again, because it is the most significant statement that I've heard from the medical field in a long time. "A cell in growth and healing mode is impervious to disease." That's huge!

As you can see, fight or flight is a necessary response to save our lives in emergencies, but should not be maintained for long periods of time. The problem is that the average person is staying in fight or flight for long periods of time. When that happens, there is one inevitable result. Eventually something breaks and shows up as a symptom. When we get a number of symptoms, we call this a disease. A disease is simply where the weak link in the chain broke under the pressure called stress.

HOW FULL IS YOUR BARREL?

Doris Rapp, MD is considered by many people to be the premier allergist in the world. She's written multiple books, especially on allergies and children. Dr. Rapp coined a theory that she called "the stress barrel." In Dr. Rapp's theory, all of us have an internal barrel that is the amount of stress we can deal with before something breaks. As long as our barrel is not full, we can have new stressors come into our lives or our bodies and deal with them quite effectively so they don't affect us negatively. Once our barrel overflows, the weakest link breaks.

When the fire alarm gets pulled, a direct message goes out from the brain to the immune system through cells that are directly connected to the ends of nerves. They are called dendrites. When I was in medical school, we were taught that these were immune cells. And indeed, they are. Then the neurologists claimed them because they give off nerve transmitters, the same transmitters that nerve cells use. So now they're called "neural immune cells" because both are true. They are part of the nervous system, and they are the direct link to the immune system. Their message is, "shut down," "stop."

IMMUNE SYSTEM ON HOLD

Why would the brain send such a message to the immune system? Well, think about it. What's the purpose of the SNS? It's to save our lives. And the immune system? What's its purpose? To fight bacteria, viruses, fungi, make repairs, and destroy abnormal (cancer) cells. Does any of that have to happen in the next 5 minutes? Of course not. Also, the immune system uses a huge amount of energy. Remember, we want all of our energy and resources to go for one purpose for the next few minutes—to save our lives! So everything that is not essential for the next few minutes gets shut down.

Well, that's fine if our immune system doesn't fight bacteria or fungi for 5 minutes, and it's fine if that food doesn't get digested for another 5 minutes. The problem today is we live in a continual state of fight or flight. As we have traveled around the world doing Heart Rate Variability testing, a fascinating and relevant phenomenon has emerged. When doing these tests, we would ask each person one question: "Do you feel stressed today?" About 50 percent would say "yes," and about 50 percent "no." Of the 50 percent that answered that they did not feel stressed, over 90 percent, when tested with HRV, were found to be in physiological stress—the kind of physiological stress that can lead to illness and disease.

I saw a bumper sticker on the back of a car the other day. It read, "If you have it, a truck brought it." Now, I hate trucks. I think these big trucks on the highway are very threatening. At least, they kick me into fight or flight. I think all of that freight should be on a railroad track. Still, I had to admit that everything in my home came on a truck—including my home itself! I actually had it built in a plant one piece at a time and hauled to the building site on a truck. If you have a health problem, it came from physiological stress—all health problems, every time.

We received a call from a gentleman who had attended one of our seminars recently. He called to tell us that after hearing this information in our seminar, he went home and did a Web search on stress. He found 67 million-plus websites that at least had the word "stress" in them. If you scan through those sites, what you will likely come away with is that if you have a health problem, it came from stress. This being true, every time you have the sniffles, any time you have an ache or pain you can't identify, if your doctor drops the dreaded cancer word on you, in short, no matter what happens to you negatively from a health perspective, you should be asking yourself, "What is the stress that caused this and how can I eliminate it?"

So why aren't we asking that question? Because up until now, we haven't had a consistent, reliable, validated way to deal with stress. What works for some people and some problems does not work for other people and other problems. The reason is that there has been a missing piece of the puzzle. And it is Secret #3 that we will get to in a few minutes.

YOUR STRESS CONTROL CENTER

Stress is controlled in the central nervous system. In particular, physiological stress is created through the hypothalamic pituitary adrenal axis (H-P-A). The hypothalamus and the pituitary were both at one time thought to be the master glands. Actually, the pituitary is a release interface with the blood so that hormones can be secreted into the bloodstream. The hypothalamus serves as a central processing unit for the whole brain. It has connections to all of the limbic system—the emotional centers of the brain. In fact, it has nerve connections to virtually every part of the brain and connects to the rest of your body through the hormones that it manufactures and releases through the pituitary. Here is a short list of some functions the hypothalamus controls:

1. Arterial blood pressure
2. Body temperature
3. Regulation of body water by thirst and kidney function
4. Uterine contractility
5. Breast milk
6. Emotional drives
7. Growth hormone

8. Adrenal glands
9. Thyroid hormone
10. Sex organ function

Physiologically, the effects of stress result in change in all of the above organs, especially in the adrenaline, cortisol, glucose, insulin, and growth hormone release.

How do we measure stress in the body? We can measure individual levels of the above; however, a test called Heart Rate Variability (HRV) has become the standard for measuring physiological stress. It is extremely valuable because it reflects the balance in the autonomic nervous system. In medical science the best tests are simple, reliable, easily reproducible and measure what you are trying to test. The Heart Rate Variability test is a beautiful example of this. In design, it is simple in that it measures the increase and decrease (variability) of the heart rate in relationship to breathing patterns. It is reliable in that it is a "gold standard" test. It is the best medical test that we have for measuring the autonomic nervous system.

The balance of the ANS equals growth and healing which adds up to health, whereas imbalance or stress in the system leads to disease and ill health. That balance is what we are able to change and scientifically measure with The Healing Codes, and The Healing Codes can do it consistently. Our commercial-grade HRV program was quite expensive when we bought it, but you can now buy inexpensive HRV testing equipment and programs for use on your home computer for under $1000 and prove it to yourself.

SYMPTOMS: THE WEAKEST LINK BREAKS

How does the body manifest stress? In what we call diseases or symptoms. Why so many different symptoms or diseases if there is only one cause? The answer is simply that we have broken the weakest link. This may be a genetic predisposition or the result of a toxin we have ingested or from prior physical injury.

Let's walk this out step by step. Let's say you have a problem with a disease by the label of "acid reflux." You experience stress. Stress decreases muscle tone around the lower esophagus, because that requires blood and energy, which we are using to fight or flee. Now the acid in the stomach washes back up into the esophagus, damaging the lining of the esophagus. These cells get repeatedly damaged, causing pain and eventually ulcers or cancer. But they only do that because they're not in growth and healing and repair mode, or they could protect themselves from the acid bath. So you manifest the disease "acid reflux."

The medical solution is to give a purple pill to stop the acid. This works quite effectively for reducing the acid, but the problem is that the acid is needed to digest food. Acid also functions to kill bacteria that we have ingested with the food. In masking our symptom, we've created two new problems. The extra bacterial load burdens the immune system. The food remains in the stomach longer until the stomach finally produces enough acid to digest it, but now there's a longer exposure period of the acid to the esophagus. It becomes a vicious cycle. So, do we want to mask the symptom or heal the source?

Obviously, we would rather heal the source, and as we have clearly shown, the source is stress.

WHAT DOES THE HEALING CODE DO TO STRESS?

As mentioned, the Heart Rate Variability test is the best medical test in existence for measuring physiological stress in the autonomic nervous system. It has been used for over 30 years in mainstream medicine and is in the same category as CT scans and MRIs, in that it does not respond even 1 percent to the "placebo effect," which basically means, "it's all in your head."

When I first discovered The Healing Codes, I looked for ways to test it because I wanted to make sure, first of all for myself, that it was "the real deal." I had been familiar with the HRV test and, in fact, had used it to test other modalities such as chakra balancing and acupuncture points—what is called the meridian system. Many people do find relief with these modalities that usually involve tapping or rubbing on acupuncture points, meridians, or chakras, but our experience was that the people got "out of balance" (which indicates stress) an hour or two after therapy.

In fact, here are the actual results. From 1998 to 2001, I did four different HRV tests on modalities using the chakra/ acupuncture points system. Between 5 and 9 out of 10 people remained in balance according to the HRV after one session (depending on the group). However, after 24 hours the number who remained in balance (normal state or lack of physiological stress) dropped dramatically—only about 2 out of 10.

In contrast, when people have been administered a pre-session HRV test, done a Healing Code, and then had a post-session HRV test, 8-9 out of 10 people were in balance after one Healing Code session (i.e., in 20 minutes or less). After 24 hours, 7-8 out of 10 people remained in balance.

In 1998 in a book titled *Stopping the Nightmares of Trauma*, Dr. Roger Callahan reviewed 30 years of use of Heart Rate Variability tests and stated that there were only two modalities cited in the literature that had been found to take the autonomic nervous system from out of balance to in balance consistently. Both of them took a minimum of six weeks to accomplish this balance. One was performed on humans and one was on dogs. Clearly, the autonomic nervous system is very resistant to rapid change. This is why it can be so difficult to change your metabolism or lose weight.

Compare this with people who have been tested with The Healing Code who go from "out of balance" to "in balance" in 20 minutes or less. This means that in 20 minutes or less the person's immune system is going from not operating the way it's designed to, to being able to function normally and able to heal whatever needs to be healed.

One of the things that so astounded me (Ben)—and other medical doctors will confirm this, along with HRV manufacturers and experts—was that our results are not only unprecedented in the history of medicine, but until we did them repeatedly, they would have been considered by many doctors to be impossible.

Although these HRV test results were not a formal study, clinical, controlled or double blind, they certainly provided a piece of evidence we needed to show open-minded people that The Healing Code can remove stress from the body in a way that is needed for long-term healing, and in a way that had never been measured before. In fact, Dr. Callahan stated that "by and large, double blind studies are to show that a treatment is making a difference, when nobody can tell if it's making a difference." If it is obvious that the therapy or treatment is making a difference and doing no harm, the need for double blind studies is greatly diminished.

Also according to Dr. Callahan, the need for double blind or controlled studies is not nearly as critical when dealing with Heart Rate Variability because HRV is not even 1 percent susceptible to the "it's all in your head" placebo effect. That is the main factor that makes double blind and controlled studies necessary—to rule out placebo. Many experts agree that using HRV automatically means that you've ruled out the placebo effect.

The other piece of "proof" was provided by our clients' actual results, which were both consistent and predictable.

Here's what happened at one conference we did, as reported from the director:

Dr. Alex Loyd and Dr. Ben Johnson were keynote speakers at our most recent PQI International Conference in Ixtapa Mexico. There were hundreds of people there from all over the world. Over a three-day period Dr. Loyd worked with 142 people who had something bothering them physically or non-physically. Dr. Loyd gave each person the appropriate Healing Code for the cellular memory connected to the thing bothering them the most. All 142 people self-reported that the memory had gone to a zero within a few minutes—a 100 percent success rate! All three days there were people laughing, crying for joy, and waiting in line around The Healing Codes booth. People even reported dramatic physical healing resulting from self-administering one Healing Code. The word miracle was the word heard most often. One lady from

Montreal, Canada who called it a miracle had remarked before doing The Healing Code that "if that memory went to a zero she would put posters of Dr. Loyd in every room of her house." As many healings like this one occurred, word spread through the conference that you could have a life changing experience at The Healing Codes booth. I think at one point they had over one hundred people on a waiting list for personal Healing Codes. Dr. Loyd and Dr. Johnson also spoke five times at the conference and we had to turn people away from several of those [sessions], as word had spread about The Healing Codes.

—Dr. Ellen Stubenhaus, PQI Board Member

This is why we say confidently that The Healing Code addresses the source of illness and disease in the body.

MANY SYMPTOMS, ONE CAUSE

Recently we had a testimonial come in from a gentleman who actually purchased The Healing Codes package for someone else. He got home, looked through the manual, and decided to try it on his own problem before he gave it to his friend. He had multiple skin lesions all over his body. In fact, he had already talked to his medical doctor about having them cut off and doing plastic surgery. He had a lesion on his forehead and a number of others on his back and one on the top of his head. He started doing The Healing Codes, and in a relatively short amount of time, a matter of weeks, the lesions had flaked off until finally, when he called us, they were all gone except the one on his head inside his hairline. By that time, about 90 percent of it was gone and he was confident it was going to go away, too.

Well, how in the world can something that physical, like multiple skin lesions, heal in a period of weeks? Because stress is at the root of this problem, and The Healing Codes heal stress. Once stress is removed, your immune and healing systems are capable of healing just about anything. Normally when we think about trying something like The Healing Codes, we think about emotional issues, but stress is at the root of every problem, emotional and physical.

Please understand: All of the physical and non-physical problems that we're talking about—diseases, mental and emotional issues, headaches, fatigue—The Healing Code does not "treat" any of those. None. Never has, never will. The Healing Code only heals issues of the heart, which reduces or eliminates physiological stress in the body.

That's Secret #1: The one source of illness and disease in the body is physiological stress, and The Healing Codes have been found to eliminate this kind of stress in the body in a way that is unprecedented in history.

WHAT THE HEALING CODES USERS SAY (HRV RESULTS)

Dr. Alex Loyd and Dr. Ben Johnson were the keynote speakers at our annual Scholars' Reunion this past year. They taught everyone The Healing Codes, did before and after HRV tests to show their effectiveness, and taught the Healing Codes advanced training material. Of the fifty people that were at the conference, there were only two who were not in HRV balance after one Healing Code session. Six of these same people retested twenty-four hours later and all six were still in HRV balance with no additional intervention. I don't think it's any coincidence that—when asked at the end of the conference to raise their hands if they had experienced physical or nonphysical healing over the weekend as a result of doing The Healing Codes—all fifty people raised their hands. There were participants with major diseases, some in great health, and just about everything in between. The Healing Codes worked for everyone.

—Bill McGrane, McGrane Institute, Inc.

I attended one of your unbelievable sessions. My HRV was so low you were concerned for me. I did only the Code you taught us then. My depression has lifted, and I have been so well I forgot about doing them. Oooooops!

—Marilyn

In 2003, I attended some training that was being done in Kansas City for coaches. At one point, volunteers were asked to come to the front of the room to be observed by the class as they were monitored by HRV while thinking about an issue that caused intense emotions. I volunteered because I had found myself to be in an increasing state of fight or flight over a business decision I had made a few weeks earlier. I was feeling extreme financial pressure at the time and the image of walking out to my mailbox to retrieve what was sure to be a stack of bills for the startup, was a trigger that had been putting me in an absolute state of panic.

The most disturbing part of this was that I had done my due diligence before making the decision, had felt very good and had even established clients for my services. I had nothing to regret at that point. I knew that the knot in my stomach and the crippling fear wasn't founded on anything going on presently.

When summoned to the front of the room at the training, I sat down on a chair. The large screen was out of my view but the people in the room were able to observe the results of my HRV. Dr. Loyd had me close my eyes and relax as he began doing The Healing Code on me with the intention of healing the pictures associated with my issue. I was pretty oblivious to what was going on in the room and on the screen. I found myself focusing on the physical feeling of anxiety and wondering if The Healing Code would work in this situation. I kept seeing that image of walking to the mailbox with a sense of dread. I was trying to keep the image out of mind so I could relax but the sense of doom and gloom was very prevalent.

An amazing thing happened. I'm not sure how long it took but I suddenly noticed that the knot in my stomach was melting away. I found my thoughts drifting to memories of other endeavors that had been successful. A sense of confidence came over me. The realization that I had initially taken the proper steps to be successful led to the conviction that I just needed to get to work and follow the plan I had set for myself. The panic I had been feeling almost seemed comical as a sense of peace came over me, because I realized how unfounded the panic was. Two days later, I was still feeling very balanced as I thought about going to the mailbox, and the HRV reading showed proof that I was still in a balanced state.

—Teri, Nashville, Tennessee[7]

7 For more testimonials, visit www.thehealingcodebook.com.

CHAPTER TWO

Secret #2:
Stress Is Caused by an Energy Problem in the Body

In 1905 a guy with crazy hair named Albert scrawled on his chalkboard $E=mc^2$ and the world has never been the same. To know why, you have to understand just what $E=mc^2$ means. On one side is E, which stands for energy. On the other side is everything else. In fact, that is the meaning of $E=mc^2$: Everything is energy and everything boils down to energy.

All our health problems originate from a destructive energy frequency. To explain how, I will ask you to use your imagination a little bit. Let's say that somehow we knew that I was going to develop a tumor in my liver in 10 days. I don't know how we know; we're pretending, okay? What if we did a little experiment and went to Vanderbilt Hospital here in Nashville to have an MRI done on me every day for the next 10 days? What would happen in our experiment? The doctor would come back with results from the day one MRI and might say, "All clear" ... on day two, "No problem"... on day three, "Why are we doing this?"... days four, six, eight, "This seems pointless"... day ten; "Oh, Dr. Loyd, we've got some abnormal cells in your liver here—we should do a biopsy and check it out."

Question: *Where did the abnormal cells come from?* We were measuring everything physical that an MRI can measure every day. The answer is that the abnormal cells *have to begin somewhere not physical!* In fact, all of your problems originate from something not physical.

Before 1905, science followed Newtonian physics, which said (among other things) that an atom is hard, solid matter. We have known for some time now that this was never true. If you look through an electron microscope that is focused on an atom and moving closer and closer to the atom, eventually you would say, "Where'd it go? What happened to it?" because the closer your focus gets to an atom the more the atom disappears, until finally you go right through it. What am I trying to say? The atom is not solid at all. The atom is made of energy. Just like everything else on planet Earth.

Everything is energy, and all energy has three common elements:

1. A frequency

2. A wavelength

3. A color spectrum

So whether it's a table, a banana, your gallbladder, or one of the elements on that eighth-grade chemistry chart, everything is energy. What type of energy something is can be determined by the frequency. Once this was proven mathematically by Albert Einstein (and, by the way, this has recently been validated by research from the Hubble telescope), everything in the world changed. Every industry you can imagine began to shift toward electronics and energy. The automobile industry, the communications industry, television, radio, you name it. The one industry that has lagged behind more than most is the medical industry. Especially in Western medicine, this industry has continued along the lines of Newtonian pre-1905 physics, despite the fact that we now know it is limited in its ability to describe the way the real world works.

When I first discovered The Healing Codes, one of the things that convinced me that this system was legitimate was my library research on what the greatest minds of our times have said when they spoke about health issues. What I found absolutely astounded me, and I had never seen it before even through two doctoral programs covering six years of my life.

What I found was that some of the greatest scientific minds of our times—Nobel Prize winners, people with doctorates in various fields, medical doctors, authors, inventors—had said, when they spoke about health issues, that the root of all health and illness is always an energy issue in the body. They also said that someday we're going to find a way to fix the energy problem that underlies every health issue, and on the day that happens, the health world will change forever.

Here are a few examples of what I found:

"All matter is energy."—Albert Einstein

"All living organisms emit an energy field."
—Semyon D. Kirlian. U.S.S.R.

"The energy field starts it all."
—Prof. Harold Burr, PhD, Yale University

"Body chemistry is governed by quantum cellular fields."
—Prof. Murray Gell-Mann, Nobel Prize Laureate (1969),
Stanford University

"Diseases are to be diagnosed and prevented via energy field assessment."
—George Crile, Sr., MD, Founder of the Cleveland Clinic

"Treating humans without the concept of energy is treating dead matter."
—Albert Szent-Gyorgyi, MD,
Nobel Prize Laureate (1937), Hungary

So if you're going to heal health issues at their root, you have to heal the energy problem. You have to heal the destructive frequency in the cells that an MRI identifies and that is interpreted by a doctor as a potential cancer cell or Parkinson's disease or whatever the problem is.

ENERGY: THE QUANTUM LEAP IN UNDERSTANDING OUR WORLD

In the past almost all energy phenomena were ascribed to the deities or some spirit being mischievous. During the Era of Enlightenment and the Renaissance periods, we began to more fully and accurately understand how things actually worked, and formed theories to describe phenomena. Scientists like Copernicus, Kepler, and Galileo challenged previous views of astronomy and celestial orbits and brought new information to light, specifically that the planets, including earth, orbit around the sun, as opposed to previous theory that they all rotated around the earth. Isaac Newton furthered the scientific enlightenment with the well-known theory of gravity he discovered when (as the story goes) he was knocked on the head by an apple. He also developed calculus and the three laws of motion. These theories all worked pretty well for what we knew at the time. However, we knew that there were a lot of things they didn't explain.

When Albert Einstein, one of the most brilliant scientists to ever live, showed that $E=mc^2$, the scientific world was launched into a new paradigm—one that much better fit what was happening in the universe. Science has taken a quantum leap with this knowledge. We have now learned to use energy in ways that as a boy I read about in the pulp fiction hero comic books. I remember Dick Tracey talking to his partner through his two-way video wrist radio—we now have cell phones that small. You could literally wear them on your wrist if that were the fad. And men going to the moon—what a fantasy! But we did it. I have no doubt that someday we will have a tricorder device like the doctor on Star Trek used and even be able to transport people from place to place using energy fields.

A MATTER OF QUANTUM PHYSICS

How can all this happen? It is called quantum physics. Quantum physics is very difficult to explain, but let me give you some examples from experiments that the Department of Defense of the United States performed.

In 1998, they scraped cells from the roof of a subject's mouth and placed them in a test tube. They hooked the test tube up to a lie detector or polygraph. Then, they hooked the subject up to a polygraph, but in a totally different area of the building. They had the subject watch different types of shows on television. Peaceful, soothing shows and violent, stimulating shows. What they found was that the individual's cells registered the exact same activity at the exact same instant as the person. When the individual watched the calm, soothing shows, the physiological response of both the individual and the cells would calm down. When it switched to stimulating material, the individual and his cells would both show physiological arousal. They continued to separate the individual and his cells farther and farther apart until finally they were 50 miles apart. It had been five days since the cells were scraped from the roof of the subject's mouth, and they were still registering exactly the same activity at exactly the same instant.

Another experiment with very similar effects, but from one individual to another instead of from the person's own cells, was called the Einstein-Podolsky-Rosen experiment. In this landmark study, they took two individuals who were virtual strangers, gave them a few minutes to become superficially acquainted, and then separated them 50 feet apart, each one in a Faraday cage (electromagnetic cage). A Faraday cage is designed to prevent radio frequency and other signals from going in or coming out. For instance, you could put an FM broadcasting antennae in a Faraday cage and 50 feet away, you could not tune your radio to that frequency and receive it because the Faraday cage effectively blocks those frequencies. In short, a Faraday cage blocks normal energy, but allows the flow of quantum energy.

Once in the Faraday cage, they hooked both individuals up to an electroencephalograph (EEG), which monitors neurological activity. They shined a penlight in the eyes of the first subject, but not the other. Shining a light in someone's eyes like this causes measurable neurological activity and visible constriction of the pupils. At the instant they did this, the neurological activity of both subjects showed the same EEG activity and pupilary constriction. They changed subjects and separated them farther and farther apart with the same results each time.

PARANORMAL PHENOMENA OR QUANTUM PHYSICS?

The conclusion drawn from that study is that we are transferring information from person to person at an unconscious level constantly with people we are connected to even superficially. For the first time this explains hundreds of validated instances of what had seemed for decades like paranormal activity. An example: A mother is having lunch with a friend of hers in New York City and at 12:15 looks up from her salad with a horrified look on her face, and says to her friend, "Something has happened to Jane … I must call Jane." She immediately abandons lunch and calls California in an effort to find her daughter, Jane. She finds that at exactly 12:15 Jane was in an automobile accident and is shaken, but okay.

I personally knew of one of these events when I was a young boy. My best friend's name was John. His parents, Marina and George, had gone on a short trip to Fairfield Glade about an hour and a half away for a quick getaway, leaving John in the care of his older sister, Tina. About halfway to Fairfield Glade, John's mother said to her husband, "We have to go home right now. Johnny's in trouble." Arriving home sometime later, they found John with his head stuck between the banister rails of the stairway, while his sister was listening to music through headphones, unable to hear John screaming. John was fine, but shaken.

So, how did Marina know that John was in distress and danger? For many decades, we chalked it up to ESP or various other paranormal phenomena. We now know, thanks to the Einstein-Podolsky-Rosen experiment, that it was simply hard and fast laws of nature called quantum physics. In the case of Jane and her mother and my best friend John, the unconscious transfer of information simply came up into the conscious thinking of the individuals involved. While unusual, this is far from unheard of. In fact, more and more people are discovering ways to access this unconscious information through the use of quantum physics for healing purposes.

This brings up the topic of mysticism, because outside of the explanation of quantum physics, these scientific experiments would appear to be mystical. What we have called "mystical" in the past is most of the time simply where someone has learned to use the natural functions of quantum physics for a particular application. Or, as in the case above, it happens by accident. There are people who can bend metal objects or move things with their minds. Or who appear to know things that they would have no way of knowing. Now, for sure, there are magicians out there, but they are not using quantum physics, they are using sleight of hand or illusion. This is not what we're talking about. The truth is simply that before now we have not understood how it could possibly happen before. As we begin to understand quantum physics, we gain insight as to how these things can actually occur. In fact, one of the benchmark theories of quantum physics is that, given enough opportunity, virtually nothing is impossible. So what we've considered to be mystical is not mystical at all, but simply quantum physics that we haven't understood because we've been operating under Newtonian theories.

AN OVERDUE PARADIGM SHIFT

Do we need to be afraid of quantum physics? Not at all. It's the way the universe functions and always has. We just haven't understood it before. As you will see later in this book, the understanding of quantum physics is opening up the greatest breakthroughs of healing and health that we have ever experienced. It's a new understanding, a new paradigm shift in thinking, but one we must make. Just think about this: If you were transported to Salem, Massachusetts, in 1692 and flipped out your cell phone and called a friend, what do you think would have happened? They didn't understand the physics of a microphone, batteries, chips, LED displays, or radio frequencies traveling through the air. You would have been prosecuted as a witch because they didn't understand physics. Is there something evil about cell phones? (My wife would say "yes.") Does that mean that the physics didn't exist? If you had had two radios back then and used them, could you have talked to each other? Of course! Physics hasn't changed, only our knowledge, understanding and application of it.

People who were the first to discover certain aspects of physics and the way the universe was created have always been misunderstood and sometimes persecuted or martyred. The list is long and distinguished. Copernicus (who discovered that the earth and other planets revolve around the sun), Galileo (who proved Copernicus' theory mathematically), Columbus (who proved the world was round), and many others were persecuted for discovering scientific truths. The sailors on the Nina, the Pinta, and the Santa Maria were all absolutely convinced they were going to sail off the edge of the earth because they believed it was flat. They believed in an old theory which not only wasn't true then, but never had been.

But don't expect to find a great understanding of quantum physics among the public or even educators. I (Ben) recently looked in my daughter's eighth-grade science book and she was being taught the same Newtonian physics that I was taught in the eighth grade forty-five years ago. The tragedy is, we knew even when I was in eighth grade that this theory was outdated. It takes an old theory years or even decades to get out of the general mindset even when it doesn't fit anymore.

Fortunately, now more and more people are coming to understand the significance of energy as described by quantum physics, in spite of its being ignored in general education.

Reviewing the principles for you is essential to comprehending the revolutionary power of The Healing Code.

THE MANY FACES OF ENERGY

Energy can take many forms. For instance, there is energy that we call "light." It encompasses a certain spectrum of the energy frequency, from $4.3 \times 1014 - 7.5 \times 1014$. We detect these frequencies with our eyes. There are sound frequencies. We detect these with our ears and receptors in our feet and body tissues. There is infrared energy. We detect this as heat. There is ultraviolet, which is just beyond what we can see on that end of the light spectrum. There are many other frequencies of energy that we have no receptors in the body to detect. These, of course, at one time were thought to be mystical, but now we have instruments that can detect them. We call these x-rays, ultrasound, radar, UHF, VHF, etc. The list is infinite.

There are three main components to frequencies. One is how many times the frequency changes from positive to negative in a given time period. We usually call this cycles per second. For instance, electricity is 120 cycles per second in Europe and 60 cycles per second in the US. There is amplitude, and that is the magnitude of the wave above and below the baseline, or zero point. Then there is the shape of the wave. That's right, waves have shapes. You can have a sine wave, which is a nice, smooth, curved, symmetrical wave that reminds you of an ocean swell. There are spike waves, which are straight up and straight down like a needle. There are square waves, and many other shapes. There are frequencies that we use to carry other frequencies. We have now figured out how to send hundreds of thousands of messages per second through a little tiny fiber using light frequency. We call these fiber optics, and we use them every day when we talk on the phone. It's all still pretty mystical to me, because I don't completely understand how it works, but do I use it? You bet!

What about medicine and frequency? Do we use frequency in medicine? Well, yes, on a very limited basis, when we have to. But understand this: When you realize what frequency is and what it can do, you understand that using frequency in medicine would literally do away with the pharmaceutical industry as we know it. Do you think they will let that happen? Using frequency for diagnosis is safe, and becoming fairly common. X-rays were the first usage of a frequency to make diagnosis. EKGs, EEGs, and HRVs are all examples of detecting energy/frequencies to make a diagnosis. Ultrasound uses sound waves in this process. The latest entrée is Magnetic Resonance Imaging (MRI). Now most people think that the significant word in MRI is "magnetic." But the magnetic field only enhances the resonance, or frequency, of the atoms to make them more visible. The whole reason MRI works is because of the resonance, or frequency, of the atoms; this is what MRI detects.

WHAT THE PHARMACEUTICAL/MEDICAL INDUSTRY DOESN'T WANT YOU TO BELIEVE

Well, what about healing? Remember, this is very "dangerous" territory. Would you take a stick and go into the lion's den and shake it at the lion? The pharmaceutical industry has more money, power, and leverage with politicians than is imaginable. The truth is, frequency has been used in healing for decades. There was a PhD in the 1920s and 30s by the name of Royal Ramon Rife who was consistently successful with cancer patients using frequency alone. He was actually the discoverer of how to use one frequency to carry another, as was just mentioned. Rife invented a light microscope that could see up to 30,000 power decades before the electron microscope. No light microscope before that could see greater than 100 power. His brilliant discoveries were apparently a threat to some people, however. His lab (with his records) mysteriously burned down, and he was denigrated as a scientist. One of the most brilliant scientists of the twentieth century died a broken derelict.

So therapy using energy frequencies has only been allowed to enter medicine where there are no effective drugs; for instance, with kidney stones. We use energy at the frequency of sound to break them up. Dermatologists now use certain light frequencies to stimulate healing and hair growth to damaged skin. The *Parade Magazine* of the newspaper reported an experimental cancer therapy where they insert a tiny needle probe into a tumor, tune the probe to the frequency of the tumor, and it burns the tumor up. So medicine is beginning to enter the "age of energy." But make no mistake, there are tremendous forces standing against this move, especially if ordinary people were to be able to use this themselves in their own living rooms. Think about the loss of power, money, and control throughout the whole medical establishment if people could heal themselves without a doctor or professional practitioner.

STANDARD APPROACHES

Let's take a look at how standard medicine currently approaches a major affliction in our society: cancer. Standard medicine's question is, "How do we kill the cancer cells?" You never hear them ask—and wouldn't it be important to ask—"What caused the cancer?" What a phenomenal question! *What caused the cancer?* Seems to be a logical question, but one I (Ben) have never heard asked from standard medicine in all the decades that I've practiced, and cancer is my area of specialization. Standard medicine's approach is, "Let's try to cut out the local manifestation of the process that we call 'cancer.'"

This is not an unreasonable thing to do for a local tumor. However, it still does not change what caused the cancer. I can't tell you how many patients that I've worked with who are on their fourth or fifth type of cancer because no one ever thought to change the "why" of what caused their cancer. If you're going to get a standard medical cure for cancer, it is almost always surgical. But again, I can't tell you how many patients I've seen in my clinic who were told "we got it all," only to have "it" come back.

Standard medicine's next approach is to kill the cancer cells. This is done with radiation or chemotherapy. They both work in similar fashion, by damaging cells. Unfortunately, cancer cells look, act, and metabolize remarkably like all of the rest of the healthy cells in your body. But not only that, cancer cells are quick learners and they rapidly learn how to defend themselves against chemo and radiation. In fact, they are much more resilient than normal cells.

Here's how chemo works: It damages the DNA of rapidly dividing cells. Cancer cells are rapidly dividing, so that's a good thing, right? Well, yes; however, there are many other cells in your body that are also rapidly dividing. Most unfortunate of all is that your immune cells are normally the most rapidly dividing cells in the body. What is the first thing a chemo doctor checks before he gives the next dose of chemo? Your white blood cells. Your immune cells. But let me (Ben) help you gain a greater understanding of the significance of the damage to the immune cells. If you were to ask an oncologist (chemo doctor) if chemo could ever possibly kill all of the cancer cells, the honest answer would be a resounding "never!" It doesn't work that way. At its very best, chemo might kill 60, 70, maybe even 80 percent of the cancer cells, but there will always be some remaining. That leads us to this thought. "If the chemo is not going to kill all the cancer cells, and if I'm going to live, what's going to kill the rest of the cancer cells?"

If your immune system cannot step up and kill the last 20 or 30 percent of the cancer cells, you will die from that remaining cancer. Herein lies the irony. Chemo destroys the only thing that can possibly save your life. Unless your immune system is able to hit that home run in the bottom of the ninth, the cancer wins. The question is, what kind of shape do you want your clean-up batter to be in, since he has to hit the home run? Please hear this: In the end, there is nothing manmade that can heal cancer. Your immune system has to finish up the job. In fact, there's nothing manmade that I know of that can actually heal any disease. I know a lot of doctors have taken a lot of credit for healing cancer, but in the final analysis, it's always the immune system that finishes the job. The immune system is always the real star.

ADDRESS THE SOURCE

So what are the causes of cancer? Ultimately it is stress that is caused by cellular memories. On a physical level there are four causes, but you'll have to wait until Secret #3 to read about these.

In general, if you want to address the source, no matter what the disease or symptom, you have to do it with energy, because energy is the source. That's one of the main purposes of this book—to let you know that there have been discoveries and applications of these discoveries that will allow you to take a good deal of your life, health, and prosperity into your own hands. Not only will you not sacrifice results, but you can achieve results that have never before been possible.

STRESS IS CAUSED BY INSUFFICIENT ENERGY

All illness and disease is caused by insufficient energy at a cellular level. Chronic fatigue syndrome (CFS) is a relatively new diagnosis as far as medical history is concerned. Standard medicine has dismissed, denied, and misdiagnosed these unfortunate souls for decades. It reminds me of the woman with the issue of blood who came to Jesus to be healed. "She had suffered a great deal under the care of many doctors and had spent all the money she had, yet instead of getting better, she grew worse" (Mark 5:26). Some things never change, do they? This is not a knock against standard medicine. There are good and bad in every type of medicine and healing I have ever found. Some truly care and want to help, and some are in it for the money.

Let me help you understand what is happening on a intracellular level with low energy states such as chronic fatigue syndrome. As we said earlier, low energy is actually the basis of all illness. You recall we talked about fight or flight, that is, stress and how it affects cells. Let's take a closer look. As the cells shut down to conserve energy in the body, oxygen isn't getting into the cell, nutrients aren't getting into the cell, and glucose (fuel for the cell) isn't getting into the cell. The power plants of the cell are being starved. These little power plants are called mitochondria.

As the mitochondria go, so go the cells. As the cells go, so goes the body. These little power plants–the mitochondria–look remarkably like bacteria. In fact, evolutionists believe that they were bacteria that established a symbiotic relationship with cellular structures in order to provide power for them. Something that we seldom think about is the effect of many medications that we take. Because our focus is relieving symptoms, we frequently forget about the details, and the devil is in the details. We have been overdosing society with antibiotics, passing them out like candy. We have known for years that almost all respiratory tract infections are viral. Antibiotics have no effect on viruses yet they are still frequently prescribed. The U.S. Federal Government has begun a campaign to get physicians to stop prescribing antibiotics unnecessarily for the common cold and ear infections.

Now remember our little mitochondria look just like bacteria. Antibiotics will frequently kill mitochondria along with the bacteria. In fact, the antibiotics that we have been giving unnecessarily may be a major cause not only of CFS, but the increase in many other diseases and new diseases as well. There was recently a study published that showed that women who had received eight or more doses of antibiotics before their eighteenth birthday had a dramatic increase in breast cancer. We can no longer turn a blind eye to the side effects of the drugs we are giving and being given. By the way, there is nothing "side" about side effects. They are unwanted direct effects of the drugs.

THE "DELCO GENERATOR" INSIDE

Our bodies are not like houses in a city, which are all connected by an electrical wire grid to one giant electrical plant. It's just the opposite. One hundred years ago, before we had electrical grids, if you wanted to have electricity you needed your own generator. We had an old Delco generator on our farm. You put gas in the tank to fuel the generator. It required a source of oxygen (air intake) and it had to exhaust the by-product in the form of fumes. As long as the fuel lasted, you had electricity.

It's the same way in our cells. A cell has to have oxygen and glucose (fuel), and it has to be able to exhaust the waste out of the cell. When you stop that process, you get a "brown out" where the cell doesn't function properly, and eventually a "black out" just as with the Delco generator when it ran out of fuel. If the process goes too far, the cell will literally die. So you can see how stress sending these cells into a state of alarm can cause an energy shortage, leading to cellular damage and what we would eventually label as a disease. The type of disease or diagnosis that manifests is simply determined by which link in the chain breaks.

A study came out in 2007 that made headlines all over the world, about the discovery of genes that make proteins that go into mitochondria. Earlier studies at Harvard Medical School and elsewhere had already ascertained that even if the rest of a cell is destroyed—the nucleus and other parts—it can still function if the mitochondria are alive. The latest discovery in 2007 by David Sinclair, a pathologist at Harvard Medical School who helped lead the research, isolated the protein that activates the genes that keep the mitochondria healthy. This has gotten researchers to dream of a "wonder pill" to fight aging. "What we are aiming to do is to find the body's natural processes that can slow down aging and treat diseases like heart disease, cancer, osteoporosis and cataracts," Sinclair said.[8]

---

8 "Wonder Pill To Fight Ageing Could Become A Reality," *Reuters*, September 21, 2007, http://gulfnews.com/news/world/usa/wonder-pill-to-fight-ageing-could-become-a-reality-1.201890.

Researchers are growing more hopeful that they can get to the source of what keeps us healthy. This is encouraging, but medicine is still far from thinking in terms of going to the source. What would *you* rather address? The symptoms or the cause? The disease or the initiating event?

We believe we have discovered the thing that does what those researchers are hoping a pill will someday do.

INTERRUPTING THE SIGNAL

How does a Healing Code intervene in the cellular process? The brain detects and sends energy frequencies telling all other parts of the body what to do. The hypothalamus in the brain sends 911 signals to other parts of the body when an emergency is present and the body needs to prepare to defend itself from whatever the emergency is. When there is not a real emergency but we are thrown into fight-or-flight mode anyway, these frequencies are destructive instead of life saving. A Healing Code changes destructive energy frequencies and signals into healthy ones. The way to change a destructive energy frequency to a healthy one or to one that is not harmful anymore is relatively simple. Here is a sine wave:

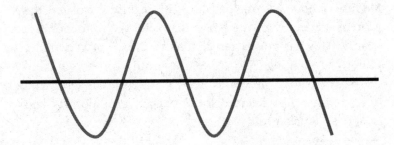

Let's assume that this is the energy frequency of cancer. The way that you change that frequency is to hit it with one that is exactly opposite. That would look like this:

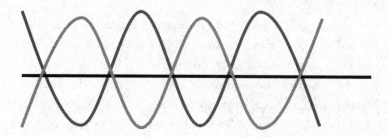

When you do that, here is what you come out with:

You have just neutralized that destructive frequency, and if you can neutralize the frequency, the source of the frequency is either healed or it will heal if you can keep that frequency neutralized. And that's what a Healing Code does.

THE PHYSICS OF NOISE-CANCELING HEADPHONES

Ben recently told me of an experience he had that was a beautiful illustration of what we have just been talking about. Dr. Ben was on his way to be filmed for the DVD, *The Secret*. He was flying from Chattanooga to San Francisco. Now, Ben hates noise. If we are in the same hotel room on a lecture tour, any little sound (that I don't even notice) would drive him crazy. Well, Ben's plane took off, engines roaring, people talking, babies crying. Before the trip, Ben's wife had given him a noise-canceling headset. So, he pulled it out, put it on, flipped the on switch, and WOW—no more noise! No crying, no roaring engines—beautiful silence! Ben couldn't believe it. He took them off, noise still there—put them back on—tranquility again!

Almost giddy, Ben went rummaging for the instructions. He *had* to know how this miracle was possible. The booklet said that there was a microphone built into the headset that recorded the outside noise. Once recorded, the headset created an exact equal opposite frequency to the noise, which cancelled out the noise. This is the quantum physics of The Healing Code in a nutshell. The Healing Code is like a noise-canceling headset, but for the issues of the heart, not noise.

The Healing Code stops the hypothalamus from sending that 911 signal when that signal should not be sent. A 911 signal from the hypothalamus is what puts your cells into stress mode; it's what shifts your blood flow away from your internal organs, your higher intellectual functioning, and your immune system, which we talked about in Chapter One on the source of stress in your body.

Another way to put this is that The Healing Code stops the hypothalamus from sending the energy frequency signal that initiates a stress response in the body when a stress response should not be occurring. How does it do that? It does that by using the body's own healthy energy frequencies (the opposites of the destructive frequencies) to overcome the destructive energy frequencies, like turning on a light in a dark room. The light always overcomes the darkness. The healthy energy will overcome the destructive energy frequencies.

Can we prove that? As we described in Chapter One, we can prove that The Healing Codes remove stress by the HRV results. Can we prove that The Healing Code fixes the energy problem associated with a problem in the body? The way we can prove that is by the testimonial results of clients who do The Healing Code. In other words, their problems go away when they do The Healing Code. The only way the problems could go away is if the destructive energy frequencies are eliminated, the hypothalamus stops sending the 911 signal when it shouldn't, the cells in stress mode open up, and the immune system is allowed to heal the way it is designed by God to heal.

So, what are some of those client results?

∽Ↄ∾

BASAL CELL CARCINOMA (CANCER)

One of my best friends is a brilliant medical doctor. When I first showed him the small growth on my arm he was not concerned. Though we were in the same weekly Bible study together, my seminar schedule and winter month clothing kept the danger "growing" on my arm hidden from his eyes for months. The first time my doctor friend saw me on a warm spring day in a short sleeve shirt I was in trouble. With one look he took me aside and said, "Larry, this is a basal cell carcinoma, you need to get it removed immediately before it metastasizes or it could kill you." The following Monday morning, before I could make an appointed for surgery, Alex Loyd called and asked if we could meet to discuss the Hebrew basis for the results he was getting with what would come to be called "The Healing Codes." We met for lunch. If anyone other than Alex had been telling me about energy healings, I would have run. Energy medicine sounded wrong to my western ears and my religious programming. After listening for a long time, I rolled up my sleeve and asked, "Are you telling me that I can get rid of this basal cell carcinoma by running my own energy back in to my body?" Alex, said, "I can only tell you the amazing results that some of my clients have experienced." My reply was, "I need a couple of days to pray and study Hebrew root words, I can't do this until I come to peace about it." Two days later, with clear insights on the physical results of "stress" in the spiritual heart, I called Alex and the rest is history. What I experienced next was absolutely amazing—to the point that I have been telling people all over the world about The Healing Codes in my "Rediscovery of The HEART" seminars ever since. I could tell a difference in the tumor in three days, I watched it get smaller and smaller day after day, it was completely gone in four or five weeks. That was over eight years ago—still to this day not a trace of the tumor has returned. I cannot recommend this process too highly. It is, in my opinion, a major breakthrough that heals any issue at its core. What the origination of the computer has done for business, The Healing Codes can do for health and healing. — Larry

∾⤳∽

THYROIDITIS, FIBROID TUMORS, GALLSTONES, EPSTEIN BARR, CHRONIC FATIGUE SYNDROME, ETC.

In August of 2003, I had been having health problems for three years. The diagnoses I had received included: Hashimoto's thyroiditis, adenomyosis, fibroid tumors of the uterus, fibrocystic breast disease, laryngopharyngeal reflux disease, a gallbladder full of gallstones, Epstein Barr virus, panic attacks and chronic fatigue syndrome. I had spent thousands of dollars on medical bills. I had tried medicine, nutrition, and supplements. I was in bed for two months and the people of my church had to bring meals to my family. I could not function in my roles as a wife and mother. I had to take a sabbatical from my work for health reasons....After doing the [Healing Code] exercises 3-5 times per day for six weeks, I experienced a dramatic healing. An ultrasound performed ten weeks after beginning the Healing Codes showed no fibroid tumors! When I questioned the doctors as to what could have caused this, one went so far as to say that the radiologist who read the ultrasounds which confirmed the fibroids for two years in a row must have been wrong. He could not explain the amazing healing. I have not taken thyroid medicine for the last year and am off of all prescription medicines. To this day, I have not had my gallbladder removed (I was told two and a half years ago that it was packed with gallstones and should be removed). I have only had one gall bladder attack since beginning the exercises and that was early on. I eat a normal diet and am doing wonderfully. My energy and strength have returned and I continue to practice the exercises daily. I thank God for His healing of my body and for revealing His healing power through The Healing Codes discovered by *Alex Loyd.* I recommend The Healing Codes to everyone who needs a physical or emotional healing. — Jennifer

CANCER, NEUROLOGICAL PROBLEMS, DEPRESSION

I was diagnosed with cancer, neurological disorders and depression. With the Code, slowly the problems went away. Our bodies are programmed to reboot like computers given the right actions. Thank you. —Anisti

CHRONIC FATIGUE SYNDROME AND FIBROMYALGIA

I was one of the most successful in the United States in my field until I developed severe symptoms and was diagnosed with chronic fatigue and fibromyalgia. After two years I was mostly bedfast, in constant pain, on numerous medications, and without hope. After doing The Healing Code exercises for six months, I am: off all medications, am totally free of an incurable disease, feel better than I did before I was diagnosed, and am working again. In short I HAVE MY LIFE BACK! — Patty

SUICIDAL DEPRESSION

Suicidal depression had forced my family to make major changes out of their fear for my well-being. I had no energy, no desire for life, and everything seemed like a mountainous chore. My husband is an MD but he was at his wit's end—we had tried everything. I was very skeptical when I heard about The Healing Codes, but I was more desperate. In less than two weeks my depression was completely gone. Not only could I not believe it—no one around me could either. Now my entire family and a number of friends do the exercises—some do them every day, some when a need arises. The Healing Code has truly been a gift from God. — Mary

NIGHT TERRORS

My son had been having night terrors for about ten years. He would wake up most nights screaming with nightmares—we would try to comfort him but he was not awake and would not wake up. Sometimes the episodes would go on for a long time—it was exhausting and very traumatic for the whole family. We tried everything from changing sleep habits, to taking special herbs, to prayer, to doctors. Nothing helped! After one Healing Code exercise the night terrors were healed and never returned—that was more than a year ago. I have told everyone who will listen to me to try The Healing Code–it works! — David

DRIVING PHOBIA AND PANIC ATTACKS

I have had a phobia of driving in heavy traffic which I treated with EFT. I found the phobia would return whenever I was in very heavy traffic, especially at night. I would go into a panic attack while driving, which is very frightening. While in Nashville I worked on this issue with The Healing Code exercises. On the way home I had to drive ten hours in heavy rain through the mountains with no visibility. I made it home without any bit of anxiety. Since then I have realized that this was not only affecting my driving, but also was a part of my life in many other areas as performance anxiety. I now find that I am very relaxed in every area of my life. — Maryanna

ABANDONMENT ISSUES

Within the few weeks I've been working with The Healing Codes, I've changed, now feeling free to talk to people and express my own opinion. That might sound insignificant for some, but for me it is a big step. I've dealt with an abandonment issue all my life, always worrying that if I say something, others might not like it and leave me, ignore me, or just not hear or see me—a fear of being invisible to others. Healing this belief makes a big difference in my daily life. —Therese

PERFECTIONISM

I struggled with perfectionism for years. Everything I said was sprinkled with disclaimers. I worried that people were always judging me. After finding a picture related to my perfectionism, I used the exercises to heal that belief. What a difference. I am not afraid to speak out and say what I believe. —Lucy

PFO (HOLE IN HEART) CLOSED UP

In September 2007 I had a TIA (mini-stroke). I had started doing The Healing Codes three months prior. I recovered quickly from the TIA, but of course they did all kinds of tests to discern the cause. They decided (from some spots on the brain shown by an MRI) that I'd had another undetected TIA, and that the cause was a PFO—Patent Foramen Ovale, or hole between the chambers of the heart. This had caused unfiltered blood to move up to the brain, which resulted in the TIAs.

Apparently PFOs used to be routinely closed up by inserting a small device to "plug" the hole. However, the FDA had decided that this procedure was no longer allowed. Medication (Plavix and aspirin) was the new protocol. Many doctors don't agree with this solution, and were trying to get the device approved again. The Director of the Stroke Program of the Neurosciences Institute at Central Dupage Hospital and the head of the Heart Hospital at Edwards Hospital in Illinois asked if I would be willing to be part of a clinical trial. I said yes, and got in the "device" group.

Meanwhile I continued doing The Healing Codes. I told the medical people that I realized they were not going to listen to what I was going to say, and they would probably think I'm crazy, but if perchance when they got in to insert the device the hole was not what they expected, I have been doing something called The Healing Codes and it's possible the hole might close up as a result. I had heard so many amazing testimonials of the results of doing THC that I knew it was possible.

Of course they paid no attention. I went in for the clinical trial procedure in January 2008. When I woke up and asked how it went, my husband told me that the hole was way too small for the device, and I was booted out of the clinical trial.

I'm sure it was an embarrassment to the medical people. But the head of the Edwards Heart Hospital, Dr. McKeever, did ask for information on The Healing Codes in my follow-up visit. He said, "In my entire career, I've only heard of three or four spontaneous closings of a PFO."

The doctors still wanted to know what caused the TIA. They figured it was arteriovenous malformations in the lungs. Tested that. Result: "AVMs were too small to be seen."

My own doctor (who has MD and DO degrees) translated for me: "Diane, that means they're not there." She got The Healing Codes, saying there's no other explanation for my story but that The Healing Codes healed me.

I've continued doing this simple protocol for more than two years now. I am off most of my medications (I was taking the Plavix and medications for asthma, allergies, overactive bladder, acid reflux). My bone density test showed added bone mass (which my doctor said was remarkable). I can go on and on about the emotional results, too, but I'll quit here. — Diane

∽◈◡

CHANGE THE FREQUENCY, HEAL THE PROBLEM

What we want you to particularly notice about these testimonials is the range of issues they cover. Everything from major health issues to relationship problems, career problems, and peak performance problems … almost everything that you can imagine.

So not only does this show that Healing Codes heal the energy frequency problems in the body, but this also confirms Secret #1—that there is one source of all health issues. The Healing Codes are a quantum physics healing system like the physicists quoted earlier have been predicting for many years. As the destructive energy frequencies are changed to healthy ones with Healing Codes, both emotional and physical issues are healed.

Why would you want to use quantum physics instead of chemicals (medicines) or nutritionals to heal a stress and energy problem? The critical factor in either approach is the transfer of information to the problem. Chemicals and nutritionals are transferred from molecule to molecule at the rate of about one centimeter per second, and a little is lost in each transfer. The transfer of information through energy occurs at around 186,000 miles per second, and almost nothing is lost in the transfer. This is why cell phones and the Internet have become so popular—they allow almost instantaneous communication that was fantasy on Star Trek thirty years ago. In the same way, The Healing Codes make possible in the body and mind what our greatest minds have foretold for the last eighty-plus years. If the origin of the problem is energy, doesn't it make sense to heal it with energy?

ENERGY TRUMPS GENETICS

I received a phone call one day from a woman in Oklahoma who told me a heart-wrenching story about how her son was diagnosed with leukemia at six months old. Christopher Ryan had probably been through more procedures, surgeries, chemo, radiation, and medications than any ten people normally go through in their lifetime. His mother, Melissa, called me in 2004 when Christopher was eleven or twelve. They were starting to see familiar symptoms in Christopher again that were very disturbing. Christopher was throwing up regularly and they couldn't seem to stop it. He had a hernia that was getting worse and worse and causing him discomfort. Christopher was tired all the time and had dark circles under his eyes. Melissa said, "We're going back to St. Jude's in Memphis, where we've been going since he was six months old, and I am so afraid of what those test results are going to show."

Well, they had twelve days at that point before they went to St. Jude's, so I immediately sent her The Healing Codes. Melissa and Christopher started doing Healing Codes that very day and did them faithfully for twelve days. Christopher started feeling steadily better. His vomiting stopped, his dark circles went away, and his energy came back. Melissa said the light in his eyes came back. By the end of twelve days Melissa Ryan was convinced that Christopher was healed.

I was doing a seminar close to their home not long after that, and at the end of the seminar this handsome young man came up to me with some papers in his hand. He said, "Dr. Loyd, my name is Christopher Ryan and I wanted to bring you my test results." Everything—MRI, CT scan, blood work, lower GI, upper GI, EEG–everything–was 100 percent clear. No more throwing up. The hernia was gone. Everything was perfect! A few months later Melissa Ryan sent us a video testimony in which Melissa is holding Christopher in her arms and fighting back tears of joy. She puts her hand on a large stack of bills on a table next to her and states, "This is over a million dollars in medical bills. What a million dollars in medical bills could not do, The Healing Codes have done."

Now how in the world could this happen with something so severe that has such a concrete physical and structural and genetic history? If you can remove the stress, almost anything can heal. We measure this stress through detecting destructive energy frequencies. When the destructive energy frequencies are gone, so is the stress. The research at Stanford and at the Institute of HeartMath in California indicate that if you can remove the stress, then even genetic issues very often can and will heal.

In this situation, an alarm frequency was being sent for some reason that was putting Christopher's body into stress mode when it should not have been. Over time this manifested as his leukemia and the other physical problems he was experiencing. The Healing Codes did not ever "treat" his leukemia, his throwing up, his hernia, his lack of energy, or any of those other issues. All The Healing Codes did was to allow him to remove the stress from his nervous system by stopping the stress signal, which is an energy frequency, from being sent. That's how Christopher's healing, which seemed like a miracle, could occur. These kinds of results can occur when that signal that should not be sent in the first place is stopped and the body's stress response is stopped. The first things stress turns off are the healing and immune systems, and when the healing and immune systems are turned back on or turned way up, they are capable of healing just about anything. The Healing Codes did not heal Christopher; he was healed by his own immune system.

UNEXPECTED HEALING

A gentleman named Joe Sugarman, who owns one of the newspapers in Maui and is considered by many to be one of the top copywriters in the world, invited Dr. Ben and me to come and lecture in Hawaii. For years, he has brought people to Maui to lecture about subjects like natural healing and health. When he started doing The Healing Codes he said to us, "You know, I've been bringing health experts into Maui to lecture for years. While I have seen miraculous results with other people, nothing has ever helped my health problem at all." His problem was chronic foot pain from an automobile accident. Joe limped noticeably, had difficulty sleeping well, and was in almost constant pain.

He asked me, "Do you think The Healing Codes can help my foot?" and I explained, "Well, you know they don't even address foot problems; they work on the cause of stress in the body." Joe started doing The Healing Codes and about three months later he wrote to us to say that within three weeks of doing them, his foot pain was 100 percent, completely gone. It was completely healed and has not come back. He also related that he had other issues he hadn't really been working on that also healed at the same time, and nothing had ever helped them before, either. The biggest thing, even bigger than his foot healing, was the wonderful emotional healing from some things that had bothered him his whole life, healing he had never experienced until he did The Healing Codes.

Now let's review where we are so far:

Secret #1: There is one source for almost all health problems, and The Healing Code heals that source, as shown by mainstream medical diagnostic tests.

Secret #2: According to the greatest minds of our time, every problem is an energy problem. The Healing Codes heal the energy problem, as proven by testimonials of healing just about any problem you can imagine by doing them.

Now, on to Secret #3.

CHAPTER THREE

Secret #3:
The Issues of the Heart Are
The Healing Control Mechanism

We told you in Secret #2 you'd have to wait to learn the source of stress. We hope you didn't skip ahead, because you missed some good information there. Now here is the answer. It is the most significant point and, indeed, is the reason why this book was written. We are going to tell you the cause of stress in the body. We have known this and have been talking about it for years, but now there is scientific validation.

It is cellular memory.

Not only was this the missing piece in the puzzle in health sciences for decades, it was my (Ben's) missing piece of the puzzle as well for my patients and myself. I've given many lectures on the causes of cancer over the years. Those causes are emotional issues, heavy metals, acid pH/oxygen deprivation, and viruses. I usually listed emotional issues last for several reasons: (1) no one wants to admit that they have any, (2) if they do, they don't want to talk about them, and (3) we haven't had a way to effectively deal with them on a medical level. Drugs only mask symptoms but don't really help. Talk therapy frequently makes it worse because it opens up old wounds that your body has been trying to heal.

There are effective ways to deal with heavy metals. EDTA and DMSA and other heavy metal chelators are pretty effective, so we can get heavy metals out of the body. Acid pH balance is tougher because it is a lengthy (months to years) process to change that balance and involves significant dietary changes, although there are effective agents now that we can use nutritionally to alter that more rapidly.

Viruses are even tougher because the little buggers can hide in your DNA. It's hard for one of your white blood cells looking for the "bad guys" to find them when they are inside of one of your own cells, in the nucleus in the DNA in the cell. But there are now effective antiviral formulas using low-angstrom silver, graviola, una de gato, and sangre de drago. There are even some anti-viral drugs that are of modest benefit.

BEYOND THE PHYSICAL

In my alternative medicine cancer clinic in Atlanta, Georgia, USA, I had ways to deal with the viruses, the acid/base balance and the heavy metals, but I had no way of dealing with the emotional issues, even though I went through a master's degree in psychology and employed a staff therapist.

I still remember the day that the importance of emotional issues crystallized in my mind. I had a sweet young woman in my clinic who had breast cancer. I had worked with her quite successfully. The tumors were all gone, according to the CT scan, the tumor markers, and the physical exam. But the patient died anyway. This woman had a significant emotional issue in her life that she could not resolve. Her husband was extremely controlling. They were actually quite wealthy, but she did not have a credit card or checkbook. She had to ask and sometimes beg for everything she needed or wanted.

However, there was one thing that he could not control in her life, and that was whether she lived or died. She chose to exert her self-control in the only way she could find.

I was looking and searching for some way to help with my patients' emotional issues when my own need arose. It is one thing when your neighbor's house catches on fire. It's terrible. When your own house catches on fire ... now that's cause for panic. As I've already mentioned in the Preface, I was diagnosed in 2004 with Lou Gehrig's disease by two doctors. I would much rather have been given the diagnosis of cancer. Eighty percent of people diagnosed with Lou Gehrig's die within five years of their diagnosis, and I, personally, do not know any ten-year survivors, although I hear there are a few. They are, however, extremely debilitated. My house was on fire, and I didn't have long to put it out. There was some good news in that I didn't have to try a lot of surgeries or drugs because there were no known medical benefits to any therapy.

An acquaintance told me about The Healing Codes and that I should go hear about them. Since my house was burning, I thought I should go investigate. I was desperate. I would consider anything.

"SHOW ME THE SCIENCE"

What I heard that night in Dr. Loyd's presentation was scientifically sound in the realm of physics. He had many testimonials of significant healing, but I've heard testimonials before. Thousands of them. In fact, on a daily basis, my patients would say to me, "Dr. Johnson, I read where XYZ cured someone of my type of cancer." To which I would respond, "Show me the science." I was willing to consider anything to help my patients get well, but I never wanted to give them false hope, and certainly not waste their money. So it was always important to see if there was any scientific basis to a claim. I was impressed. Dr. Loyd had actually validated his methods scientifically with Heart Rate Variability studies, the gold standard medical test for physiological stress in the body. I had to try The Healing Codes.

As mentioned earlier, within six weeks of beginning The Healing Codes, my symptoms had all resolved. Two months later I went to the neurologist and he placed needles in my muscles to detect the firing patterns that are so familiar to Lou Gehrig's patients. There were none. From a medical perspective, this kind of recovery is unheard of. As I write this, more than five years later, I'm still symptom free.

CELLULAR MEMORIES: THE KEY TO HEALING

So what was this perfect code? This incredible technique? Actually, we were not even focusing on the Lou Gehrig's disease at all. We were focusing on a few cellular memories from my childhood, the kind that all of us can relate to. There were no huge traumas in my life. I was never sexually abused, I was never beaten, and I can promise you I never missed a meal. I had a pony. A teddy bear. My parents never got divorced. They didn't fight. (Now, I do have to say that, of course, I was terribly abused by my big brother and sister, who would never admit to it—just kidding, Dan and Ann.) Yet I still had "bad programming" that was sending stress signals to my cells and causing disease.

Not coincidentally, Southwestern University Medical School, Stanford University Medical School, Harvard Medical

School, and New York University Medical School have all released research indicating that these types of cellular memories may very well be the missing piece of the puzzle in health and healing. The research from Southwestern concludes that our best hope for healing incurable illness and disease in the future may very well lie in finding a way to heal cellular memory, and that "the potential is there for a much more permanent fix" if we find such a solution.[9] Why do they say this? Because it appears to be the healing control mechanism of every cell of the body.

So what is a cellular memory? It's a memory stored in your cells. Which cells? All of your cells.

For many years, science believed that memories were stored in the brain. In an effort to determine where in the brain, they cut out just about every part of the brain, and guess what? The memories were still largely intact! Even though memories can be stimulated from different areas of the brain—pleasure memories recalled when a pleasure center was stimulated, for example—the actual storage place for the memories appeared not to be confined to the brain.

Then where are they stored? The answer may have first been found when medicine started doing organ transplants. There are many documented cases where people who received organ transplants would start having the thoughts, feelings, dreams, personality, and even food cravings, of the organ donor. Today many scientists are convinced that memories are stored in the cells all over the body, not localized in one particular place.

Cellular memories resonate destructive energy frequencies and create stress in the body. Southwestern University Medical

9 "Cell Decision," by Sue Goetneick Ambrose, *The Dallas Morning News*, September 13, 2004.

School released a landmark study in September of 2004 where they reported that the healing control mechanism in the body may very well be its cellular memories—not only for humans, but for animals and plants. What did they find in the lab at Southwestern that causes them to say this? They found that as the cell memories of the organism go, so goes the health of the organism. A person, animal, or plant with destructive cellular memories will struggle even in good circumstances. With healthy cell memories, a person can thrive even if their circumstances are not ones where you would expect someone to excel. The analogy Southwestern used when they released this research is "the cell memories are like little Post-it notes that tell the cell what to do—only when there are destructive cell memories the Post-it's are telling the cell to do the wrong thing."[10]

CELLULAR MEMORIES AND "ISSUES OF THE HEART"

According to Dr. Bruce Lipton, the "wrong thing" that the cell is told to do is to go into stress mode when it shouldn't, and it is wrong beliefs that initiate the body's stress response. These wrong beliefs are imbedded in cellular memories that make up the unconscious and conscious mind, along with the control centers of the brain. The conclusion of the Southwestern University Medical School research, which was published in the *Dallas Morning News* and then reprinted all over the country, is that the future of healing illnesses and diseases that are now considered to be incurable may very well lie in finding a way to heal cellular memory.

These cellular memories and wrong beliefs are the same thing Solomon was talking about more than 3,000 years ago.

---

10 "Cell Decision," by Sue Goetneick Ambrose, *The Dallas Morning News*, September 13, 2004.

It's the issues of the heart that are the source of every issue (problem) you can have in your life—physical, relational, and even success and failure.

The Institute of HeartMath has for years done some of the best alternative clinical research in the world. One study they did definitely falls into the hard-to-believe category, but it's true. They placed human DNA in a test tube, had the test subjects hold it in their hands, instructed the individuals to think painful thoughts–in other words, recall destructive memories. It's impossible to think painful thoughts without recalling destructive memories. After the individuals did this, researchers took the DNA out of the test tube and examined it. The DNA had literally been damaged. Next, they put the same DNA back in a test tube, had the individuals hold it in their hands again, and this time instructed them to think good, happy thoughts. Again, realize it's impossible to do this without accessing good memories. They took the DNA out of the test tube, examined it, and discovered there had been a healing effect on the DNA. What does this mean? It means that the activation of certain memories appears to damage the DNA, while the activation of healthy memories may literally heal the DNA. Wow.

Dr. John Sarno, professor of clinical rehabilitation medicine at New York University School of Medicine and a physician at New York University Medical Center, contends that chronic pain and various other illnesses are caused by repressed anger and rage in the unconscious mind: "You do not know you have this inside you because you are not conscious of it." This anger and rage, which are rooted in our cellular memories, are the very things that the Institute of HeartMath found that damaged the DNA in their experiment.[11]

In 2005 on *Good Morning America*, Charles Gibson interviewed Lonnie Zeitzer, MD, from the UCLA Children's Hospital in a story that was also carried by *USA Today* and the *ABC Evening News*. In the study at UCLA, they had discovered that children's chronic pain and illness can be caused by anxiety from the parents. In other words, stress in the parents created destructive cellular memories that ended up manifesting as stress in the children. In the conclusion of the study, Charles Gibson remarks that debilitating childhood illness seemed to be caused by psychological, non-physical factors, to which Dr. Zeitzer agreed. The research involving cellular memory keeps pouring in.

WHY POSITIVE THINKING DOESN'T HEAL CELLULAR MEMORIES

One question you may have after reading the results of the study at the Institute of HeartMath is, "Well, can I just think happy thoughts and heal all my cellular memories?" I'll go ahead and tell you that the answer is unfortunately "no," because there are mechanisms in the unconscious mind that protect those memories from being healed. But we're getting ahead of ourselves. We will discuss this in more detail in Secret #4: The Human Hard Drive.

The fact that our memories are the control mechanism for our health has been the basis of psychology for at least one hundred years. This idea started to be scientifically

---

11 For an insightful interview on Dr. Sarno's theory, visit the site http://www.medscape. com/viewarticle/478840. He is the author of *The Mind body Prescription: Healing the Body, Healing the Pain*; *The Divided Mind: The Epidemic of Mindbody Disorders*;, and *Mind Over Back Pain*.

validated when our young men came back from WWI with wounds, even though they had not been physically wounded. They called it being "shell-shocked." This was the first time we realized that what is in the mind can make you physically sick.

Talking about memories may remind us of counseling and therapy, which frequently involves having to wallow in all that old garbage again. Some of you may think, "That's going to make me depressed and bum me out," or, "I'm tired of dealing with that stuff." A lot of men may say, "I don't even want to go there at all." With The Healing Code, you don't have to. Just like Joe with the chronic foot pain, you can do the Healing Code on whatever is bothering you the most and allow it to heal those cellular memories for you. Even more important than the healing of Joe's foot was the transformation of his emotional life, but note—he had not focused on it.

To have permanent, long-term healing, you have to heal the destructive cellular memories. This just makes sense. We all have memories in our lives that are full of feelings like anger, sadness, fear, confusion, guilt, helplessness, hopelessness, worthlessness … the list is endless. It doesn't make sense that any of us can have all of that inside and not pay a price. The price is our health, relationships, career, etc. We all need to have the *source* of our problem healed, not just the symptoms. Why? If you only heal the symptoms, the problem is likely to come back, or maybe two in its place because the thing that caused the symptoms is still there. The source of the problems that you want to change, that we asked you to think at the beginning of this book, is destructive cellular memories.

Once you understand this, how do you find the cellular memories that are related to whatever your problem is? Secondly, how do you heal them?

WHY "COPING" MAKES THINGS WORSE

Again, psychology has been trying to find a way to do that for decades, but some of the latest research indicates that talking about the problems over and over can actually make them worse.

The Healing Code heals the destructive cellular memories automatically. It does *not* heal cellular memory by training you to think about your problem in a different way, which is called "reframing." It does not heal by balancing your brain chemicals because chemical imbalance is a symptom, not the source of the problem. It does not heal by having you think about something else whenever problems bother you. No—I call all of these things "coping." Coping means the problem is still there, you have just learned a more constructive way to deal with the pain. What everyone really wants is for the pain to be gone. The Healing Code is a literal physical mechanism in the body that, when turned on, changes the energy pattern (Secret #2) of the destructive cellular memory (Secret #3) to a healthy one. When this occurs, the stress response of the body is turned off or down (Secret #1). This doesn't mean you don't have the memory anymore; you do, it's just not destructive anymore.

Here's the problem: *coping equals stress.* Since every problem known to man can be traced back to stress, a mechanism for dealing with our problems that creates stress is counterproductive, to say the least, and crazy to say the truth. Let me explain.

Our bodies and minds have a list of things that have to be done every day, and a certain amount of energy to do them. For the things that have to be done, there are "have to's," "need to's," and "want to's." The "have to's" would be breathing and your heart beating. The "need to's" are things like digestion, waste removal, blood cleansing, and immune functioning. "Want to's" are things like repair work, resolving old destructive memories, and the like. If the body's available energy is reduced, then things on the list have to be cut. The less serious things are cut first, which almost *always* includes the functions of the immune and healing systems.

Guess what? Keeping destructive memories suppressed requires a huge amount of energy, and it's constant. Those memories have to be suppressed every hour of every day, so you may have a significant percentage of the energy needed for living your life constantly being consumed for nothing more than suppressing cellular memories. If you're already ahead of me and guessing that this is probably going to mean health, relationship, or career problems, let me applaud you. You're exactly right. In fact, Dr. John Sarno, professor at New York University Medical School whom we've already mentioned, confirms from his research that adult chronic pain and chronic health problems result from the suppression of destructive cellular memories. The process of suppression creates constant stress, until eventually something breaks. Dr. Sarno's work, like that of Southwestern University Medical School and Stanford University Medical School, agrees that healing these memories, rather than suppressing them (which we call "coping"), results in the healing of the health condition.

According to all these sources and more, what is desperately needed, and what will change the face of health forever, is a way to heal the destructive cellular memories as opposed to merely coping with them for a lifetime. For decades we believed that coping with these memories was somehow allowing us to sidestep the destructive effect. Recent research proves that this was a deadly miscalculation. Cellular memories cause destruction whether they are consciously remembered or not.

WHAT HEALING MEANS

Once you've healed the memory, what will this mean to you? This will mean you will not feel the negative beliefs, anger, frustration, resentment, guilt, hopelessness, and other destructive emotions.

Can we prove this? Absolutely. The proof is that consistently, predictably, and usually quickly, people report to us that their destructive feelings and beliefs heal. As we do seminars all over the country, it happens in every single seminar. We have it on video, and in all kinds of testimonials—people who do The Healing Codes tell us that their feelings, beliefs, fear, anger, resentment, all those negative emotions, heal quickly and consistently. It's not at all unusual for a person to be doing The Healing Code and to tell us later that an issue they have had with a family member going back ten, fifteen, twenty or more years healed in a few minutes to a few days. They frequently tell us of all the things they tried over decades of their lives without getting the results they desire. Why is this proof? Because the destructive feelings and beliefs we experience come from our memories. The only way they can heal is if the memory they come from heals.

A woman I'll call Amanda purchased The Healing Codes® and called me to relate her experience with the system. She'd had an emotionally abusive situation with her mother. Her mother was extremely critical, negative, perfectionistic, and harsh. In short, when she was a girl, my client ended up feeling worthless, incapable, and fearful about most any situation. She became a perfectionist because of the underlying belief that she would only be loved if she got everything right (as is usually the case with perfectionists).

Amanda's life was a mess. Even though she had had great success in beauty pageants, she felt ugly. Even though she was a terrific cook, she felt that everything she cooked had something wrong with it, even when everyone else raved. When things were good, they weren't good enough, and disaster might be around the next corner. When things were bad, it was a confirmation of what she knew would happen. She would be so exhausted from work that she couldn't wait for a vacation, but after the first day of the vacation, she couldn't enjoy the rest of it because she was afraid of the vacation ending in six days.

Amanda didn't like sex for several reasons. For one, she didn't have the perfect body, so rejection was sure to come (though it never did). And why would she want to get that close to another person, anyway? Letting someone get close is just going to make it hurt worse when things turn sour. She was depressed and filled with anxiety. Confusion was a constant companion. She would often become paralyzed about where to eat lunch. She blamed herself for all of this. After all, she'd never been abused or beaten or raped or any of those terrible things, and everyone else thought her mother was terrific. None of this changed the fact that she was living in a terrible prison of her feelings, thoughts, and beliefs.

When Amanda came to The Healing Codes, she came after decades of counseling, therapy, inner exploration, religion, medications, nutritionals, self-help seminars, personal growth seminars, infomercial packages ... you get the idea. She said that when she got The Healing Codes, the one thing she felt had already been resolved in her life was her relationship with her mother, at least as far as the childhood events were concerned. After all, she'd spent tens of thousands of dollars and years of her life to get to the place where she could work a steady job, have a marriage and family, and have a fairly adjusted life. The surprise was that when she started doing The Healing Codes, the thing that kept coming up over and over and over was the childhood stuff with her mother.

The Healing Codes are not counseling and therapy, and no, you don't have to go back and dig up your past. However, as the memories are healing, sometimes we become aware of which ones are healing. That's exactly what happened with this woman. After about a month of doing The Healing Codes, Amanda's negative thoughts, feelings, beliefs, anxiety and perfectionism were gone. Zapped! Disappeared. She called to ask me if it had ever happened before that someone had spent the kind of money and effort she had and honestly felt that an issue was healed, when in reality it had not been healed at all. That they had not been healed before was obvious to her while doing The Codes. When those memories came into awareness as they were being healed with The Healing Codes, she would feel a corresponding lightness or healing or relief–something that let her know they were being healed. When a month had gone by, she could tell they'd all been healed. I congratulated her and laughed at her question about whether it had ever happened before, not to belittle her question but simply because what she described is what happens to most people. It's the exception when it doesn't happen.

COPING IS NOT HEALING

You see, we tend to confuse coping with healing. When I did private practice counseling and therapy, healing almost never happened, but I was good at teaching people to cope. In fact, that's what most counselors and therapists are trained in. Just about every self-help program I've ever seen is full of coping mechanisms. What does that mean to the person who uses them? It means that you're going to have the garbage of your problems the rest of your life, but learn to spray perfume on it every time it stinks. You're going to try to get to the place where it doesn't bother you as much. I've even heard of some counselors or therapists who say to their clients after they've learned to cope, "Your problem is healed." After all, they are the experts, so most people tend to believe it. If the problem is truly healed, then every problem that's being caused by it will also heal, and as you've already seen in this book, these underlying cellular memories are the source of physical health problems. So if healing has truly occurred, then everything should heal—not only the emotions, feelings, and beliefs, but the physical problems which were caused by them as well.

The proof that The Healing Code heals these cellular memories is in people telling us over and over that their feelings and beliefs and attitudes and thought patterns heal while they do it. We actually have a way in The Healing Codes® system to measure that, and people tell us over and over and over, using that measurement tool, how those cellular memories are healing in their lives. It's no accident that as those cellular memories heal (Secret #2), the cellular energy problem heals and people report that their health problems melt away.

We have now completed the first three secrets, so let's review for just a second.

Secret #1: There is one cause of illness and disease, and it is stress. The proof that The Healing Code heals stress is in unprecedented Heart Rate Variability results, which is the gold standard medical test for measuring stress balance in the autonomic nervous system.

Secret #2: Every problem is an energy problem. If you can heal the energy problem, you can heal whatever the resulting life problem is. The Healing Codes is a quantum physics healing system that changes energy patterns in the body. The proof of that are the testimonials from people relating that their problems have healed, including everything from major diseases to relationships to career and success issues.

Secret #3: Issues of the heart (called many things by modern science—cellular memory, unconscious, subconscious, etc.) are the control mechanism for health. They can resonate destructive energy frequencies and create stress. The Healing Code heals destructive cellular memories as evidenced by the healing of destructive feelings, beliefs, attitudes, and thoughts.

How does all of this fit together? Issues of the heart (Secret #3) cause destructive energy frequencies (Secret #2). Destructive energy frequencies (Secret #2) create stress (Secret #1). And stress is the one source of all physical and emotional problems (Secret #1).

So if you can heal the issues of the heart, you can heal just about any problem in your life. The Healing Codes heal cellular memories. Remember William Tiller's quote: "Future medicine will be based on controlling energy in the body." The Healing Codes are the fulfillment of that prediction. They are a quantum physics healing system that finds and heals destructive energy frequencies in the body.

Knowing that issues of the heart control our health is helpful. But there is more to the puzzle. "Great, there are cellular memories, but how do I get to them? How do I heal them? Where are they?"

That leads us to Secret #4....

CHAPTER FOUR

Secret #4:
The Human Hard Drive

The hard drive of your computer is where everything is stored. In fact, you can only use your computer up to the capacity of your hard drive. All of your word files, your letters, your documents, your emails, etc. are recorded there. Even when you delete a file, if you take it to a computer expert with the right equipment and the right knowledge, he or she can usually still find that file.

Inside the human computer, everything that ever happens to you is recorded in the form of memories. This is freshman psychology. Even if you can't remember it consciously, even if you were never conscious of it in the first place when it happened because your attention was somewhere else, it is still recorded. There are many documented cases of people under hypnosis or people during brain surgery who, when certain areas of the brain were stimulated, remembered things all the way back to the womb—things that were never conscious or have not been conscious for a long, long time.

Of all these memories that we have—all the recordings of everything that has ever happened to us—over 90 percent are what would be classified as unconscious or subconscious, meaning that they're either very difficult or impossible for us to remember. These would include your birth, your first bath, and the time you were just learning how to walk and knocked over one of mom's glass vases that broke on the floor. Around 10 percent of the memories are conscious, meaning that we can recall them if we try. These would include not only what I had for lunch today, but my tenth grade birthday party, when I got my driver's license, my first date, when I married my wife, my child being born … events like that.

THE 90 PERCENT BELOW THE WATER LINE

In psychology, this relationship between our recorded memories in the conscious and unconscious mind is often illustrated as an iceberg, as you see below. The iceberg represents 100 percent of our memories. The 10 percent above the water line represents conscious memories, while the 90 percent under the water line represents unconscious or subconscious memories.

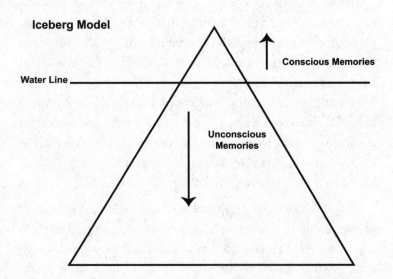

Iceberg Model

Water Line

Conscious Memories

Unconscious Memories

For the purposes of this book, we will call the unconscious and subconscious memories the "heart." I believe that actually the heart is our unconscious mind + our conscience + our spirit.

MEMORIES—WHERE AND WHAT THEY ARE

As we have already said, science used to believe that these memories were stored in our brains. The latest research seems to indicate that these memories are stored in our cells, literally all over our bodies. These memories are not flesh and blood; they are stored in our cells as an energy pattern. This is why we can't find them in any tissue of the body—they do not exist as physical tissue. Remember from Secret #2 that Albert Einstein proved with $E=mc^2$ that everything boils down to energy. Well, that includes our memories. The substance of the memory is an energy pattern, but the actual memory is an image.

According to Pierce Howard, PhD, in his book, *The Owner's Manual for the Brain*, except for people blind from birth, all data is stored inside our memories as images. These memories are also recalled as images.

Rich Glenn, PhD, in his book, *Transformation*, also asserts that all data is stored in the form of images and that a disruption in the body's energy field can be traced back to a destructive image. Dr. Glenn goes on to state that the healing of the destructive image creates a permanent healing effect in the body. Understanding this is vital to healing the cellular memories discussed in Secret #3.

Antonio Damasio, MD, PhD, head of the neurology department at USC, says, "The ability to display images internally and to order those images is a process called thought ... imageless thought is impossible ... human reasoning is always imagistic."[12]

Dr. Bruce Lipton further explains how the body is like a camera. Whatever the environmental signal is, it's picked up by the lens. The camera sees something. The lens picks it up and translates it into the film where you make a complementary copy. The camera always makes a complement of what is found in the environment.

"The truth is, in biology it's the same thing. The cell is like a camera. Whatever is in the environment, the membrane is like a lens, it picks up the image and sends that image to the nucleus where the database is. That's where the stored images are.

"The bottom line is this. When you open your eyes, what is the image you see?"[13]

The point is that what you see externally, or think you see, is largely determined by how you are already programmed internally.

DESTRUCTIVE ENERGY PATTERNS

All data, everything that happens to us, is encoded in the form of cellular memories. Some of them contain destructive, wrong beliefs that cause the body's stress response to be activated when it shouldn't, which turns off the immune system and causes literally every problem in our lives that we know of. The substance of these cellular memories is a destructive energy

---

12 Antonio Damasio, *Desccartes' Error: Emotion, Reason, and the Human Brain*, Penguin, 2005, pp. 89, 98.

13 Bruce Lipton, *The Biology Of Belief* DVD.

pattern in the body. The practical way that these are stored in the body is in the form of images, and they're also recalled in the form of images.

Let me show this to you with a very simple example. Relax for just a second and let's try a quick learning experience. What happens when you think of Christmas? Don't you remember either one Christmas or little snippets from several Christmases? And how do you remember these things? Do you see something? Do you see people's faces, a Christmas tree, or presents in your mind's eye?

Let's try it again. What happens when you think of disappointment? Don't you remember some disappointing events in your life? And how do you remember them? Do you see them? Even when you can't see a picture in your mind, you can usually recall and describe colors, shapes, objects or other visual elements. In fact we can't do anything that we don't have an image for. Before we do anything we image it, whether it's making a cup of tea, going to the restroom, or planning a city. The substance of every idea is an image, and what is the substance of an image? Is it tissue or bone or blood? No, the substance of memories and images are an energy frequency. Images are the language of the heart.

This little exercise is tapping into either your conscious or unconscious mind and recalling memories. Yes, you see them, but don't you also feel a little something? When you thought of Christmas did you feel joy? Did you smile a little bit even though you didn't realize it? Did you remember a wonderful, warm time in your life? Did you smell bacon cooking or pine scent or eggnog or cinnamon? When you recalled the disappointment memory, didn't you feel a little tightness in your chest or a little bit of discomfort?

As the research out of the Institute of HeartMath that we discussed in the last Secret proved, if you continue to think about the painful memories, the sad memories, the depression memories, the angry memories, and you focus on those for an extended period of time, you will not only feel bad emotionally, but it will literally start to send your body into the stress response we talked about in Secret #1, and over time it could literally make you sick.

THE PROBLEM BELOW THE WATER MARK

With your conscious mind, you can choose whether to think about the good, happy, healthy thoughts and memories, but with your unconscious mind, you can't really choose what you're going to think about, because the unconscious mind has a mind of its own. The unconscious mind works by association, so when you thought of Christmas, and if you have some very negative memories of Christmas, your unconscious mind could re-activate one of those negative Christmas memories, and you could start to feel bad and not even know why. This happens all the time.

I hear from people every day who say things like, "I have a quick hair-trigger anger and I just don't know why, but I've had it for a long time." Or, "I'm sad, and I cannot figure it out; I don't know why." Or, "I seem to sabotage myself at work when I'm in line for a promotion. I just seem to be my own worst enemy, and I don't know why." The reason these things happen is that you have unconscious memories that are being re-activated, and you are feeling the emotion of that original memory. Obviously, this can cause problems in your life. We're going to explore this a little bit more in Secret #5.

In Secret #4, the central fact is that everything that has ever happened to you is recorded. Some of it you can access, and we call this the conscious memory. Some of it you can't access, and we call that the unconscious or subconscious memory. These memories are encoded in the form of pictures or images, and the thing that kicks in the stress response of the body are the pictures that contain a wrong belief. As Dr. Lipton puts it, a wrong belief "causes us to be afraid when we should not be afraid."

So if you're one of these people who has wondered for years, "Why do I get angry when I shouldn't? Why do I eat when I shouldn't and when I don't even really want to because I'm trying to lose weight? Why do I think things that I really don't want to be thinking? I want to be thinking about good, healthy, positive things! Why can't I seem to break this problem involving my thoughts, feelings, and behaviors?" The issue is on your hard drive.

DEFRAGGING THE HUMAN HARD DRIVE

On the human hard drive what we're dealing with is cellular memories, and it can become contaminated with fragmented files. The Healing Code is a way to defrag our human hard drive without counseling, without therapy, without drugs, and without medications. It is a system that has been in the body forever but was only discovered in 2001. It is not acupuncture or mudras or chakras or yoga or any of those methods. It is an absolutely new discovery that has been tested with the mainstream medical tests we talked about in Secret #1.

Because whatever problems you have inside of you right this moment exist as images, as energy patterns, and the only way to heal them is with another energy pattern. Remember these statements from Secret #2?

"Future medicine will be based on controlling energy in the body."
—William Tiller, Nobel Prize Laureate

"Body chemistry is governed by quantum cellular fields."
—Murray Gell-Mann, Nobel Prize Laureate, USA

"Diseases are to be diagnosed and prevented via energy field assessment."
—George Crile, Sr., MD, Founder of
The Cleveland Clinic, 1864-1943

When you do a Healing Code, it heals the destructive frequencies and allows the wrong beliefs that are encoded into these cellular memories to heal. The Healing Codes heal that cellular memory, heal its destructive energy pattern, and allow us to believe the truth so that we are not afraid when there's nothing there to be afraid of. Then we've fixed the thing causing the problem at its source. We have defragged the human hard drive. We have healed the memories. That is what Healing Codes do, and that is why it's such a revolutionary thing. We've never had a way to do this before. The average Healing Codes exercise takes about 6 minutes, so we're not talking about something that's difficult to do or takes a long time. You can even do an exercise lying in bed or in a recliner. We've had people tell us they do them at the drive-through window while they're waiting for their hamburger. We don't advise this, but it is that simple.

In fact, Mark Victor Hansen—the co-author of the *Chicken Soup for the Soul* books who has come out publicly and said he believes that this may very well be the solution to the healthcare crisis in America—told us that he felt the biggest problem we would have in convincing people to try The Healing Code is that it's too simple. It's so simple that people just won't believe it can make a meaningful difference in their lives.

My teenage son got the flu about two weeks ago. He said he was feeling bad, and I told him to go do a Healing Code on himself. A couple of hours later he felt completely normal. Ben's daughter has been doing The Healing Codes on herself since age seven, totally unassisted. That's how simple it is!

Let's review our secrets so far:

Secret #1: **Stress is the cause of all illness and disease.**

Secret #2: **Everything is energy.**

Secret #3: **The issues of the heart control health.**

And you now know Secret #4: **All memories are energy stored and recalled as images, and 90 percent of them are unconscious.**

So defrag your human hard drive and change your life in the process. Whether you do it with The Healing Code or not, if you're going to have permanent, lasting results for your life, you are going to have to find some way to heal these cellular memories, these issues of the heart, that are causing the problem.

CHAPTER FIVE

Secret #5:
Your Antivirus Program May Be
Making You Sick

Most of us have an anti-virus program on our computer, and so does the human hard drive. So does the conscious and unconscious mind. So does, especially, what I call the heart (unconscious mind + conscience + spirit). We are born with an anti-virus program that is meant to protect us from both physical and emotional harm by ensuring that we avoid experiences that will hurt. As we have more and more negative experiences, the program adds more and more "virus definitions," just as your computer's anti-virus program does when a new virus becomes known.

The anti-virus program on the human hard drive is a stimulus/response program. Basically, it is the instinct to seek pleasure and avoid pain, and it develops more and more definitions and distinctions as we live and learn. Children don't use logic to the degree that adults do, so they operate much more on a pain/pleasure principal. If an adult is very kind and speaks in a very gentle tone and smiles at a little baby, that's pleasurable, and the baby will tend to be attracted to that person. If you let the baby take a little taste of ice cream, you will see this look come over the baby's face saying, "What's that? I want more of it!" We all have early memories like that. The opposite is also true, whether the pain is not getting the pleasure we want (like not getting the ice cream) or whether it is literal pain (like touching a hot pan). Kids learn from the pleasure or pain whether to seek or avoid something.

However, we know as adults that a child's reactions are not necessarily logical. The child may seek the pleasurable thing— the ice cream or the candy—until they're sick. Or they may avoid pain to the degree that they can't even enjoy life because of being so worried about a bug that bit them once. As adults we may also realize that not all of our own reactions are really logical. What we may not see is that in every case we too are behaving according to a stimulus/response/seek pleasure and avoid pain system.

HIDDEN SOURCES OF OUR RESPONSES

The reason we can't easily identify that our actions are responses is that we may be totally unaware of the stimulus that caused it. The stimulus is always a memory, but there are three types of memories encoded into our memory banks (hard drive) that we may not be able to recall at all. Even when we can, our response doesn't always seem logical.

Inherited memories, pre-language and pre-logical-thinking memories, and trauma memories become a stimulus/response protective programming belief system.

First of all, let's take a look at these three types of memories.

INHERITED MEMORIES

All of us inherit cellular memories from our parents, similarly to a person who receives cellular memories from the donor of an organ. I (Ben) believe that these cellular memories are literally encoded into the DNA of each cell. When a sperm and egg come together at conception, they create one cell that is a beautiful, miraculous harmony of a man and a woman. This is true physically, yes, but also non-physically. So, just as the inherited DNA is passed down that causes Johnny to have his mother's eyes and his father's chin, Johnny also receives cellular memories from both Mom and Dad.

Now, just a little bit of logic would tell you that this process also occurred when Mom and Dad were first conceived. So does that mean that little one-celled Johnny is also receiving cellular memories from Grandma and Great-Granddad and Great-Great-Great-Great-Grandmother on Mother's side that lived way before the Civil War? Absolutely. In fact, it's my (Ben's) opinion that these cellular memories are passed down through the DNA of the white blood cells in particular. Now one-celled little Johnny has everything in him that will someday grow into twenty-five-year-old Johnny, the handsome man on his wedding day. That's easy for us to relate to physically, but not so familiar in the discussion of cellular memory.

These inherited cellular memories are good, bad, and, yes, ugly (for you Clint Eastwood fans)—and everything in between. The answer to the million-dollar question that you may have is "Yes." Great-Great-Great-Great Grandmother's cellular memories can be reactivated inside of me and cause unwanted thoughts, feelings, behaviors, and physiological stress.

Don't be discouraged. If you feel like your mental pond just got a little murky and your feelings of choice and control seem to have slipped from your fingers, there is more than hope! Inherited cellular memories can be healed just like any others by using The Healing Code, as we will discuss in detail later on. I would be remiss to not state, however, that without The Healing Code, this issue can become a frustrating, and at times almost impossible one to deal with. The fact that a person's thoughts, beliefs and behaviors can be springing from something that is not even in their lifetime is irritating at best, and can lead to hopelessness, despair, and disease at worst. We believe this is one of the reasons counseling and therapy have been largely ineffective for a high percentage of people through the years. You can't deal with a problem that you don't even know exists. Fortunately, we have developed a type of testing to find these memories even if they are not remembered.

PRE-LANGUAGE AND PRE-LOGICAL-THINKING MEMORIES

Before we were able to think very rationally or talk very well, we had many events occur in our lives. All these memories are recorded just like any other memory, but they are recorded through the reasoning level of the person at the time it's experienced.

In fact, within the first six years of life, we live in what's called a Delta Theta brainwave state. This means that our experiences are "directly hardwired" into our brains without being filtered through the more rational, conscious judgment we develop later on.

If a baby wakes in the middle of the night with wet, cold, dirty diapers, he will want to scream as loudly as he needs to get the nasty feeling to go away. However, if every time he wakes his mother she is rough and angry and perhaps even hurts him, after a while the baby will also want to avoid being treated so hurtfully. He won't know anything about how hard the mother works and how miserably tired and depressed she is, because he is too young to know those words or have those concepts. He will only know that if he avoids one kind of pain (irritating diapers), he will experience another kind of pain (an angry mother). He will also feel that he has a right to be clean and dry, and a right to be treated gently by his mother, but he won't understand those emotions because he has no words or concepts for those either. All this confusion will be stored as a pre-language memory, though, which may be triggered every time he should be able to ask to have his physical needs met. Or every time he thinks of seeking comfort and love from a woman. Or even every time he wakes in the middle of the night, especially since he experienced the same negative situation over and over.

"POPSICLE" MEMORIES

I had a client one time who had an IQ of 180, had graduated from an Ivy League school with honors, and was tabbed for greatness on Wall Street. She said she didn't have any health issues, but did have success issues: "I keep sabotaging myself in my career. Everybody says I should be a mover and a shaker on Wall Street, but every time I'm getting close to something like that, I find a way to mess myself up." What she discovered through the process of doing The Healing Code was that it all went back to a memory when she was about five or six. It was a summer day and her mother had given her sister a popsicle, but would not give her a popsicle.

You may be waiting for the rest of the story: the popsicle was thrown and hit her between the eyes and she fell backwards and hurt her head really badly and they had to take her to the emergency room. But no—none of that happened. That is the whole story: Her mother gave her sister a popsicle but would not give her one. In fact, her mother even said, "Your sister has already had a good lunch; when you have a good lunch you can have a popsicle too." So what did the mother do wrong there? Absolutely nothing. But that memory was encoded through the mind, through the eyes, and through the reasoning of a five-year-old—remember, she was in a Delta Theta brainwave state at that time. And this is how the memory stays. It gets hardwired into the unconscious with the reasoning of a five-year-old throughout life until something changes or heals that.

These pre-language and pre-logical-thinking memories can really become a bugaboo (that's a clinical term) to us throughout our lives. And we have thousands of these. How much of what we know about the world is learned in the first three or four or five years of our lives? A ton of it, and all of that is encoded through the eyes and the reasoning of the age when it occurred. All of it gets recorded in that Delta Theta brainwave state, without benefit of higher reasoning.

Whenever those memories are reactivated, it will reactivate back at five months or five years, not as a thirty year old thinking rationally about it.

TRAUMA MEMORIES

These are encoded, of course, throughout our lives, whenever a trauma occurs. We can inherit trauma memories, as well.

An interesting thing about trauma memories is that when we go through a trauma, even a small one, our higher rational thinking is disconnected to some degree. Why? Because the person goes into some degree of shock. If you have seen a person in shock (even a depiction on TV) you may remember that the person may not be able to speak, may not know where they are, or may not know what has just happened. Let me explain what is going on with this process of trauma: I got a speeding ticket about four years ago and I decided to go to the school rather than have it stay on my record. That night the State Trooper welcomed us and started a little speech, and I'll never forget something he said. He said that if you are following a certain distance behind someone in normal driving conditions at night and an animal runs in front of them, and they slam on the brakes, you do not have enough time to think, "Oh, that car in front of me is slamming on the brakes. I'd better take my foot off the gas and put it on the brake and push the brake, or I'm going to run into the back of that car." You just don't have enough time to do that and avoid a wreck. However, he said, fortunately we have a mechanism that is built into us that does all this automatically. When you see those lights in front of you, your logical brain will be bypassed and it will go to your reactive brain. Your reactive brain will react immediately, way faster than you can think about it; it will cause you to put your foot on the brake, and you will not have an accident.

I don't know if that State Trooper had ever had a psychology class, but he was exactly right. This is especially relevant to things that are stored by our minds as traumas. The example of the little girl whose mom wouldn't give her a popsicle— that event was definitely a trauma to her. That may not make rational sense to us because the mother did nothing wrong, nobody yelled or screamed, there was no hitting involved, she didn't lose her house or have to move ... none of the things we normally think of as trauma happened.

What did happen, and what was encoded at that five-year-old reasoning level, is: "Mom gave my sister a popsicle, but she won't give me a popsicle. That must mean that she loves my sister more than me. If she loves my sister more than me, it must mean that there's something wrong with me. So when I'm with other people, they're not going to love me either, because they're going to realize there's something wrong with me." This became a deep-seated feeling in her and a self-fulfilling prophecy. It became hard-drive programming. "I'm not going to be loved, I'm not going to be successful, because there's something wrong with me." And guess what? That's what she lived throughout her life until she went back with The Healing Code and healed that memory.

Once my client healed that popsicle memory, she received the promotion that had been eluding her and started becoming a "mover and shaker" on Wall Street. The relationship with her mother, which had always been strained even though no one including her knew why, was healed and she became closer to her mother than ever. Everything in her life turned around because there was now nothing holding her back.

That popsicle memory was a trauma to her. At least it was to the five-year-old version of her. When anything in her life happened that was related to this memory, she felt, thought, and acted on the basis of the trauma. What are some things that might be related to the popsicle memory and therefore reactivate it? Being around other people; relationships, thoughts or conversations about success or failure, worthiness or unworthiness; just about any type of competition; food or drink; asking anyone for anything. In fact, it was hard for her to do anything that was not related. When a trauma memory is reactivated it does just what that State Trooper said: It bypasses the logical mind, and kicks in the reactive mind.

WHEN THE UNCONSCIOUS MIND TAKES OVER

What is that process called? It's called a stress response! This is what Dr. Lipton talked about regarding why people are afraid when we should not be afraid. This keeps us from performing the way we are capable of. It prevents us from being in loving relationships the way we want to. It closes our cells and eventually causes health problems.

Whenever one of those trauma memories is reactivated, the conscious thinking mind is bypassed. The unconscious mind kicks in and does whatever it needs to do. That usually involves activating the body's stress response. That is why so many times we say things or do things that work against what we really want in our lives, and we do it over and over, and we don't know why we're doing it.

These memories—inherited, pre-language and pre-logical thinking, and trauma memories—become a stimulus/response protective programming belief system.

This system is a protective system. What does this mean? It means that the mind uses these memories to protect that baby so that the baby will be able to grow up and become a man or woman. As you might expect, because this is a protective system, the pain memories are given greater priority by the control systems of the body. Whenever one of these pre-language, trauma, or inherited memories is a pain memory and something in our circumstances reactivates it, we re-experience it while our logical thinking is diminished. But what would re-activate a memory like that?

One summer when my youngest son, George, was about a year old, we had the mother of all thunderstorms. Seventy mile per hour winds were causing things to fly sideways through the air. Everything in our yard that was not attached blew away. There were a couple of tree limbs that were hit by lightening and fell with a crash to the ground. Hail, huge thunderclaps, lightening all around—it was one of those thunderstorms that's scary for an adult. The worst part of this experience is that we got caught out in the middle of the storm. Even when we were back inside our house a transformer was struck by lightening and our power went out. So George did not even feel safe when we got to the place that was supposed to be safe. It traumatized George, and this is exactly what the mind of a one-year-old is supposed to do. Why? So that he doesn't stay out there in this storm (or the next one) and get hurt. It makes him scared so he will run to safety. When this storm is over, the memory is stored as a trauma so that George will get out of the next storm that could hurt him.

For at least a year and a half afterwards, if there were any clouds in the sky George was scared and sometimes would start to cry. If the wind blew too hard, if it rained, if there was a little bit of thunder—you get what I'm saying. If any of the parts of that storm that had traumatized George a year and a half before occurred in his current circumstances, George would cry and scream. Was that logical and reasonable based on the current weather conditions? No, but George still felt what he felt during the original storm when he was a year old.

That's the way this protective programming system works. Whenever something in our current circumstances occurs that the mind associates with a trauma, the original trauma is re-activated. The mind works by association, especially the unconscious mind.

I've just told you a great secret that hardly anybody on earth knows. When you do things that you really don't want to do, think things that are really not what you want to think, feel things that you certainly don't want to feel, you have a memory that is being reactivated. Your protective programming system is making a determination that somehow the circumstance you are in is related to a trauma, possibly to your own "popsicle" memory.

THE HEART KNOWS ONLY THE PRESENT MOMENT

These are the issues of your heart—and to your heart, they are not in the past, they are happening right now. The heart is 360 degree surround sound present tense reality—all the time. So when a pain or pleasure memory is reactivated, you are not dealing with something that happened ten, twenty or thirty years ago—it is an emergency happening right now. Isn't that how it feels? Yes, it is! The thing that doesn't make sense is that it doesn't seem to fit your current situation or circumstances. So you are thrown into a state of confusion and conflict. What you feel is very strong and demands attention, but doesn't seem to make sense with your life right now.

When faced with a situation like this, what usually happens is we rationalize to keep from going crazy. We assign our feelings to something happening now, that still doesn't fit or feel right, but at least it makes more sense than anything else we can think of. The woman in the popsicle story had no idea why she kept sabotaging herself. She thought it must be because she wasn't assertive enough—so she took training courses. That didn't work, so she figured it must be something else. She's a woman, or there was something in her personality, or whatever. She kept searching for some reason to explain why she was sabotaging her success.

When we do this, it now starts a whole new problem. Now we have messed up something in our present-tense life that may not have been a problem at all, by assigning guilt to it. And worst of all, we are now believing a lie, which is the source of every problem in the first place. That's exactly what makes every issue of the heart an issue.

The last point of this secret is that your protective programming is actually a belief system. This belief system, by the time you get to six or eight or ten years old, contains deeply encoded beliefs based on memories for just about any issue you can think of: parents, relationships, identity, how threatening strangers are, how good am I at things, whether I am going to be able to succeed or fail, whether I am a good person or not, whether I am a person of worth or not, whether I am secure or not, whether I need to be afraid or can I live my life in love and joy and peace?

This protective programming belief system can have an enormous impact on the way that we live our lives. Why? It is not based on rational reasoning.

LOGICAL MIND BYPASSED

When these trauma memories occur the rational brain is bypassed and the reactive, emotional brain, the pain response brain, the stress response brain, is engaged. When these memories are reactivated, our conscious, rational thinking is either turned off or greatly diminished. So whether we are twenty, forty, or sixty years old, when that "popsicle memory" that happened when we were five years old is reactivated by something that happens today, we will not be able to deal with the situation rationally. This happens to many people all day every day. Our ability to logically think something out and reason about it and then do what needs to be done is either turned off or vastly impaired. Many people who do not live the life that they want to live are in a constant state of confusion that comes from having their logical, rational mind turned off or down because these old trauma memories are being constantly reactivated by current circumstances. These memories and this memory belief system become hard drive programming in our human computer. Pain memories are prioritized over any other kind of memory in order to allow us to survive and grow up.

The greater the pain when the original pain event occurs, the more adrenaline is released, and the broader the determination of what is identified as a similar situation later. In other words, the bigger the trauma is when it happens, the more likely it is to be reactivated later by a greater number of associations.

For example, one client kept having an old trauma memory reactivated, and one of the interesting links we found to why it was reactivated was that when the original trauma occurred, there was someone else there who was wearing a yellow tie. It had nothing to do with the trauma. They were just wearing a yellow tie. Later in life as that trauma was still affecting my client, every time he saw the color yellow, he would feel this panicky feeling, anxiety, depression, confusion, wanting to go hide or go beat somebody up. Imagine how many times a day he would see the color yellow. For sure, when he would go into his closet in the morning. Traffic signs or lights, paper, yellow pads … he'd see it everywhere. You can hardly get through an hour in a day without seeing a color like that. That trauma was so strong that this person's mind had decided that anything even remotely like this pain event must reactivate it so that he'll be on alert, because if this one happens again, he may not be able to survive it again.

This is an over-reaction of the mind. It's a case where the anti-virus program is making the person sick. But that situation with the yellow tie is not unusual at all. It happens all the time, I'm convinced, with many of us and we don't even know it's occurring, and we don't know why we're feeling what we feel or doing what we do.

GETTING AT HIDDEN MEMORIES—WITHOUT PAIN

When it comes to healing these memories, how do you do it? The traditional way is to talk about it. But I don't believe that works, and a lot of the latest research out of science and psychology indicates that talking about these memories very rarely heals them and often makes them worse. Besides, many memories are unconscious.

What most people learn to do, whether it's a memory they're aware of or not, is to cope with it. I had a client who called me and said, "My whole life is falling apart. I'm calling you as a last resort. I had a friend of mine who was healed of some physical problems working with you." She said right up front, "I don't think this is going to work. I was raped three years ago, and I've been in counseling and therapy ever since. When it happened I was healthy and happy. Today I'm on all kinds of medications, I get sick all the time, I'm about to lose my husband and children because I'm about to get divorced, and I cannot be around anybody at all most of the time. I can't give and receive love anymore the way I need to, even with my children." This person had been talking about this memory for three years with people who were highly trained, and I'm not at all saying they were doing anything wrong. I'm saying most of the approaches to deal with trauma just flat don't work. They don't have the power to heal something like that.

Why? Because our trauma memories are protected from being healed by our mind. Let me say that again: Our trauma memories—a lot of these inherited, pre-language trauma memories—are literally protected from being healed by our unconscious mind. Now why in the world would it do that? It's very simple. The unconscious mind greatly resists allowing those kinds of memories to be healed, because the unconscious mind makes an interpretation that it is unsafe for that memory to be healed, because the purpose of the memory is to protect the person from being hurt.

In the case of the woman who came to me with the rape memory, wonderful people had tried everything, and she had not gotten better. Instead, she was about to lose everything important to her, including her health and her family. She did The Healing Codes for it, and in little more than a week the memory was completely healed. At first, when I gave her a Healing Code she didn't want to do it, it wouldn't work, it was silly, it was too simple, etc. She did it; she called me back in three days; there was no change. I gave her the next Healing Code for that problem, and she called me back in three more days. No change, everything is still the same. I told her, "I don't want you to think about this memory while you do your Healing Code, but if it changes, and you'll know if it changes, just let me know. This is not counseling and therapy, and we don't even want you thinking about those things.

The Healing Codes will heal them automatically." She called me later that day and was just weeping, the kind of weeping where you're gasping for air because you're sobbing so hard. When she could finally talk a little bit all she could say was, "It changed, it changed, it changed."

When she calmed down I said, "I think you're trying to tell me the memory changed," and she said, "Yes, it did." I asked how it had changed and she said, "I was doing The Healing Code this morning and all of a sudden I recalled the memory of the rape. For the first time, I looked at the man who raped me and I felt forgiveness, and all of the anger and rage and bitterness and resentment was gone." It was replaced with forgiveness and compassion. The memory was completely healed. She reconciled with her husband, her health issues went away, she quit taking all of her medications, and to my knowledge is doing wonderfully and is happy to this day.

Her unconscious mind greatly resisted this memory being healed because it was so painful to her that if it ever happened again, she might not survive. She might have literally committed suicide or developed a terrible disease.

SNEAKING PAST RESISTANCE AND DECEPTION

If the mind resists healing these kind of memories, how are you going to heal them? The five year old's popsicle story was just about as severe to that little girl as the rape was to this adult. Now, you're saying, "Loyd, you're nuts! How in the world can you compare that popsicle story to the rape?" Because it was stored as it was seen through the mind and reasoning of a five year old, and the beliefs that became part of that memory—"I'm unlovable, there is something wrong with me, and in the future when I'm around other people they will not love me either, and I will always fail because there is something wrong with me"—those things became just about as devastating to that grown woman as the rape memory was to the adult woman.

Very different events, one we would consider a trauma, one we would not. But they were both encoded as traumas and the mind resisted healing both of them because those memories were there to protect the women from those things happening again.

A last, important thing I'm going to say about this Secret is that when these memories are reactivated—these protective programming stimulus/response memories—we tend to assign the emotional reaction we have to current circumstances. Let me give you an example. Even though the woman with the popsicle memory told me when she called, "I always find a way to sabotage myself," she had a laundry list of how everyone in her life had messed up and she believed that was the reason that she had not succeeded more. Way down deep she kind of knew that wasn't true, but at the time she always had good reason: "They don't treat me well enough … they want me to work too many hours … that person had it out for me from day one …" even when she didn't have any good evidence for these things.

The woman who was raped did the same thing: "I can't be intimate with my husband anymore because he won't be honest with me about how he sees me now." I talked to him, and he saw her just fine. He saw her as his wife who had had a terrible thing happen to her, but he wanted to put it behind them and still be intimate with her. Yet she was totally convinced that he did not see her the same way. She believed that he saw her as dirty and flawed and that he really didn't want to have anything to do with her. None of that was really coming from the situation. It was coming from her memory of the rape, but she assigned it to the situation with her husband. In other words, both women found things in their current circumstances that they could blame their reactions on, even though it was really coming from three years before, or even twenty-five or thirty years before.

Let's review Secret #5:

Inherited memories, pre-language and pre-logical-thinking memories, and trauma memories become a stimulus/response protective programming belief system.

The stimulus/response system is activated when situations similar to a trauma memory occur in the present. How broad the definition is of what is similar depends on how painful the original cellular memory was.

When the stimulus/response system is activated, the person re-experiences aspects of the original events. She experiences the thoughts, the feelings, and very possibly even the behavior. As with the rape victim, a person will feel the original feelings of rage, terror, anger and fear. She will also tend to have those thinking patterns, "This is horrible, this is terrible, I'm in danger...." She will have similar behaviors: "I want to get out of here ... I will fight to get out of here." The person will tend to assign all of these reactions to current circumstances even if it doesn't make any rational sense. She will find an excuse, a way to twist whatever is currently happening so there will be something to blame the reaction on. Even if everybody around the person knows that her reaction doesn't make sense, and even if she knows that herself, it is still what she will tend to do. She will do this because she doesn't know where it's coming from. She doesn't know that these powerful feelings and impulses come from early memories, or even if she does, she doesn't know which ones. The person has to have a reason or she will go crazy, or at least feel crazy.

In other words, your anti-virus program is functioning effectively if it keeps you out of violent thunderstorms, but it may need some re-programming if it sends you running indoors on a sunny day when a few puffy clouds float overhead.

This is exactly why so many people spend thousands of dollars and decades of their lives trying to overcome their wrong programming and live the life they desire. However, this will almost never happen by using willpower to change symptoms. You must address the source, and there's only one—the issues of the heart.

CHAPTER SIX

Secret #6:
I Believe!

In the last chapter, we talked about how the stimulus/response system sets up a belief system that is formed early in life. As our brains develop, a second belief system is formed (with language and reasoning abilities) based on the stimulus/response belief system.

When I was about ten years old we had a special assembly one day in school. Unlike some of the other assemblies we had, it was mesmerizing, inspirational, and fabulous. A karate master shared secrets of life while he did all sorts of amazing feats like breaking boards, bricks, stones, huge chunks of ice, and fighting off many attackers at the same time.

He told us a true story that has stayed with me ever since. It was of a young boy in China about my age who was in the initial stages of learning a certain form of martial arts. The school he attended would periodically have an event for the families and friends of the students to celebrate their progress. Different students prepared far in advance to do their particular demonstration. The master told this one young boy that at the event he was to break a certain number of a certain type of brick. This task was a little bit unusual since the boy had never done it before and would not actually perform the action beforehand! Yes, he would practice like everyone else, but would only practice the *technique*, not the actual breaking. When the young boy expressed concern to the master, the master simply smiled and said, "You will have no problem. You know everything you need to break the bricks."

The day of the event came and all the students performed brilliantly to the audience's delight and appreciation. Finally, for the finale, the young boy came out, bowed to the crowd, bowed to his master, and attacked the bricks as he had practiced. To everyone's amazement, the bricks broke easily under the boy's hand. The master stepped forward, motioned for everyone to be silent, and explained that what the young boy had just done had never been done before in history. Not by himself, not by any of the great masters of the world. The master shared that the boy, while talented, had been able to accomplish this seemingly impossible feat not because of talent, but simply because he believed he could perform the feat with no doubts in his heart. The breaking of the bricks was simply the physical manifestation of the boy's internal beliefs.

What are the bricks in your life? Whatever they are, chances are they are there because of a belief problem. The one thing I will promise you is that if you can believe the truth, the bricks that are blocking your path will fall away.

What this young boy accomplished many years ago in China is a perfect representation of the power that is created through believing, to the degree that almost nothing is impossible.

BELIEFS—CONSCIOUS AND REAL

The first date I ever had with my wife, Tracey (now called Hope), was in 1985. I picked her up, we went to a local park and put a blanket on the ground, and we talked for four straight hours. We talked about what we believe. We talked about life, about children, about family, about God, about religion, about everything that we could think of to talk about. I remember saying many times that night, "I think" and "I believe," and I remember Tracey responding, "Well, I believe *this*," about whatever issue we were discussing.

This was a pretty typical conversation during our dating and engagement period. In fact, I was determined that my marriage was going to be different from so many marriages I knew of that ended in either divorce, apathy, or constant disagreements. I was determined that when Tracey and I got married it was going to be because we believed and wanted the same things. I wanted us to know the potential land mines that might come up and be prepared for them. In other words, we would have a great marriage because we loved each other, had the major things in our lives in common, and were as prepared as we could possibly be.

On the day that Tracey and I got married I can honestly say that I thought we were about as ready as anyone could ever be. Not only had we had many conversations like that one the first night, we had been through pre-marital counseling, taken personality assessments and compared them, written down what we wanted in life and what we didn't want, and how we would handle certain situations. Boy, were we ready!

So we got married, and less than a year later, both of us wanted a divorce. What in the world happened? I now know that when Tracy and I said "I believe," we were talking only about what we consciously believed, what we, when looking at the logical facts, had come to the conclusion made the most sense. The problem with this is that 90 percent of our beliefs are unconscious. Our rational, conscious belief system is built on top of the Secret #5 stimulus/response protective programming belief system, and that system is largely unconscious. Even though those protective programming beliefs are locked inside our unconscious mind being reactivated whenever similar circumstances occur that could in any way potentially cause us pain, we are not aware that this is happening. So when we say, "I believe," we are saying, "I believe consciously."

After we got married, circumstances happened for both of us that reactivated pain memories which bypassed the conscious beliefs that Tracy and I had agreed on. In other words, our conscious beliefs were largely out the window, and we were living based on our stimulus/response beliefs but didn't even know it. We would assign our thoughts, feelings, and behaviors to current circumstances. I would blame Tracey and she would blame me. We would get upset, we would pout, we would do all kinds of things thinking that it was the circumstance happening right then that was the issue. But all along, it was the thing in our stimulus/response belief system that was causing the problem.

HABITS AND WHAT WE REALLY BELIEVE

Let me give you another more recent illustration of this in the area of things we call "habit."

For years, an irritating issue between Tracy and me had been making our bed. For whatever reason, that is one of my jobs, only (as you have probably guessed by now) I wasn't raised to do that. So for years in our married life, if I didn't make the bed, Tracy would become irritated and frustrated with me, which would make me feel guilty and irritated as well. I would often find myself unconsciously doing things to manipulate Tracey to make the bed herself, things like getting up a little bit later than I should have so I could say, "I'm sorry, I'm going to be late for work and can't make up the bed." I knew Tracey would make up the bed after I left. As you may have recognized, what I called "manipulation" was actually a lie. Most people lie regularly, but would never admit that and oftentimes don't even recognize it because they are so used to it. In our case, this bed-making thing had been a source of pain for both of us for a long time. After the discovery of The Healing Codes and the cleaning out of many of our destructive memories, an interesting thing happened: I didn't mind making the bed. But guess what? Tracey didn't mind now, either! No guilt, no anger, no frustration. No record keeping.

So why this story? The source of our destructive habits are heart memories. To heal them successfully, without creating more stress by coping with them for years, you have to heal the destructive memories that are the source of the habit. When you do that, the issue heals automatically and, in most cases, effortlessly.

An interesting note here is that the experts in the field of breaking habits focus almost exclusively on conscious behavior and thinking. This is like pushing a rock uphill to end in a vicious cycle—a cycle that can end up consuming decades of your life, and all this work yielding only temporary results. In the case of alcoholics, most people are aware of the cycle of quitting for a while and then falling off the wagon. This is true of all habits, but ones with chemicals involved present another barrier that has to be overcome.

ADDICTIONS AND THEIR SOURCE

Somehow or another, I've worked with a number of professional wrestlers. One had good results and the word spread. I remember one situation where a wrestler flew into Nashville to see me and shared his dilemma with me. He said that Vince McMahon, head of WWF, had called him into his office recently. Vince said he already had two strikes against him for substance abuse. If he got a third one he was out. This giant of a man—who, by the way, was one of the nicest men I've ever met—told me that his current choice is either to be a professional wrestler who makes six to seven figures a year and has action figures at Wal-mart—or to work at Wal-mart. He had tried inpatient, outpatient, all the popular books, programs, pills, therapies—you name it. He was desperately fighting for his life and his family. Over the next two days, he did intensive Healing Codes. He didn't work on his addiction, but rather on his destructive cellular memories that were blocking the addiction from being healed. He flew home addiction free. I saw him in Orlando, Florida, four years later, and he is working, healthy, happy, and still addiction free.

It has been common knowledge for years in the field of mental health that women with eating disorders believe something about themselves that is not the truth. In fact, everyone else knows it's not the truth. The amazing thing is that these precious, beautiful women can look into a mirror and their wrong belief is so strong that they will literally see a different body than the one that is there. Other people can stand right beside them in front of the mirror and they can even point to the same body part at the same time, but the anorexic person will see a distorted version of what is in the mirror. This is one of the clearest examples of how destructive heart pictures in general, and destructive stress-response beliefs in particular, can cause us to view the world in an untruthful way. Yet, we can be 100 percent convinced that our belief is accurate.

What most people don't understand is that this phenomenon happens on a continuum from being totally deceived, like the anorexic, to viewing the 100 percent truth. In other words, most of us view our world inaccurately to some extent every day. I've heard a relative of mine, who has always struggled with weight issues, say a number of times when passing a mirror, "Something must be wrong with that mirror. I know I'm not that overweight." In other situations, I've heard the same person remark, "This outfit doesn't fit me right. It makes me look overweight." Now, to everyone else in the family, the truth has been obvious for decades. There's nothing wrong with the mirror. The outfit does fit. She's overweight! This is the same principle as we saw with an anorexic, just to a less destructive extent.

BELIEF AND PERFORMANCE

A whole other way to view these belief problems is in the area of sports and peak performance. The other night I was watching the NBA finals. The commentators were talking about players who want the ball when the game is on the line, and players who don't. They described the difference as being that the players who want the ball believe they're going to make the shot, while players who don't want the ball believe they will miss the shot.

The commentators are exactly right. I remember being told a story about Michael Jordan. Often before games, he would spend time visualizing what might happen during the course of the game, including taking that last-second shot that determined who won and who lost. When it came to the actual end of the game where the outcome hinged on the last few seconds, Michael did want the ball. I've seen several interviews where he shared that in that situation, he believed he was going to make the game-winning shot.

I went to college on an athletic scholarship in tennis. Even then, this same mechanism was common knowledge among tennis players. We called it "iron elbow," that critical time in a match when one swing could mean the difference between victory and defeat. Some players would play their best at these moments and almost always win. Other players would be in such fear that they almost literally couldn't swing their rackets. It was as if their elbows had turned to iron. If you watch virtually any major sporting event for very long, when it gets down to "money time," you will hear commentators and players alike saying things such as: "When it gets to that point of the game, it's all mental"; "It comes down to heart"; "Who wins or loses at the end of the game is not about the physical anymore, but the mental"; "It's all about heart when the game is on the line."

YOUR BELIEFS CAN HEAL OR KILL YOU

Our beliefs are not only relevant to the ball game, the recital, the play, and to anorexia, they are relevant to every area of our lives. Whether our relationships are intimate, passionate, and fulfilling is determined, just like with Tracey and me, by our beliefs. Whether you are a six-figure performer at your career or in a constant state of eking by in frustration is determined not so much by your abilities as by your beliefs. Please note that if your beliefs are loving and truthful you will develop exceptional abilities in whatever your area is. More on that in Secret #7.

Let's revisit the popsicle story for a moment. That woman had all the ability in the world: 180 IQ, Ivy League training, and a mind geared toward financial matters. Everyone around her said that she had the tools not only to succeed, but to excel. In spite of this, she had become a chronic underachiever and was finding new ways, literally every week, to sabotage her career. Every single time, she could come up with a rational reason for these mess-ups: "I had a cold," "One of my assistants didn't finish what she needed to," "A friend of mine has been going through some things that have distracted me," "My cat has been sick," "So and so has it out for me," and on and on and on. Are all of those issues she brought up lies? No! Those things did bother her. They'd bother anybody. The thing that was ruining her life did not have anything to do with any of those excuses. It was the wrong belief she had from the popsicle event when she was five years old that her mother did not love her as much as she should and so there must be something wrong with her.

Ultimately, because these things kept happening over and over, year after year, she finally came to the conclusion that something else must be going on. That's when she called me. It had been a belief problem all along. When we fixed the stimulus/response belief that was causing the problem, her rational conscious belief automatically changed. Did she still have daily things that did not go her way? Of course. We all do. But now she blew right through them like a hot knife through butter, and all of those abilities started to blossom into what everyone had predicted for her—greatness.

Want to hear something wonderful? That is what is intended and predicted for you, too. Greatness. When you get your beliefs to line up with the truth, that's just what will happen in your life, too.

It's not a coincidence that the research at Stanford University Medical School found that the trigger for illness and disease in the body is always a wrong belief and, conversely, that once we believe the truth and keep believing the truth, our cells become impervious to illness and disease. What you believe will kill you or heal you.

FINDING HIDDEN BELIEFS

How do you know if you're having a stimulus/response belief that's being reactivated and that the problem is not your current circumstance? There are several very simple ways:

1. Your feelings. If your feelings do not match your current circumstances, then you can almost be guaranteed that you are having an old stimulus response pain memory that's being reactivated. However, most times you won't be aware of this reactivation happening. The feelings will be so real you will think that it's your circumstance, even if everybody else sees clearly that it doesn't make sense. So ask a friend. Say, "Here's the situation, and here's what I'm feeling about it. Is this logical for this situation, or is this a little bit extreme? And please be honest with me. Please don't tell me what you think I want to hear; tell me what you honestly think."

2. Your thoughts. If the thoughts you're having about your current circumstances are totally logical, and other people also see them that way, then you probably do not have a stimulus/ response memory that's being reactivated. If, on the other hand, your thoughts are not in harmony with your current

situation, then you are having a pain memory reactivated. We want to be living in the present, not the past or the future. Surprisingly, very few people can do this. The reason is that painful cellular memories are being reactivated that cause thoughts and feelings from the past.

3. *Your behaviors.* If you do things repeatedly that you really don't want to do and that work against your life purposes, you are acting upon a stimulus/response memory. A very obvious example is weight issues. We have so many people who come to The Healing Codes and want to lose weight, and they usually do. But when you see people who want to lose weight and continue to overeat, you can be guaranteed that they are having cellular memories that are being reactivated. They assign it to current circumstances ("I'm under a lot of stress, I'll quit tomorrow…"). You've heard this if you haven't used it yourself. The reality is that almost any addiction or destructive habit becomes locked in by painful cellular memories. The beliefs in those cellular memories are being reactivated and causing pain. The addiction is used to numb the pain or to try to feel good for a few hours.

4. *Loss of conscious control.* The most popular way of dealing with all these problems is what I call "coping." If you have a health issue, it's treating the symptom instead of addressing the source. Sometimes you can push that rock up the hill for a while … you can manage … you can cope … you can do better … but it's always a forced struggle. You often feel tension as you try to stay on the straight and narrow. That tension is stress, and that tension can end up harming you. That's not the way to do what you want, feel what you want, and think what you want. The only way to accomplish this is by healing the cellular memories.

So if your rational belief system is not taking you where you want ... if you're sabotaging yourself ... if you just seem to be unlucky all the time ... if you keep having nagging or severe health problems ... if your relationships are not the loving, intimate, joyful, peaceful relationships that every one of us desires ... if you are not able to live what you rationally, logically believe from looking at the facts ... it is because your stimulus/response belief is being activated, causing you to react to old pain just like you did when that memory originally happened. In short, you end up living a life that's not the life you want to live.

WHAT YOU DO IS WHAT YOU BELIEVE

We always do what we believe. If you're doing something wrong, it's because you believe something wrong. One hundred percent of what we do, we do because of what we believe. You're ready to punch me in the nose, right? You say, "I've done tons of things in my life that I shouldn't have done, knew at the time I shouldn't have done, felt bad afterwards, and there was a bad result." You're thinking, "I violated my beliefs in order to do that!"

Respectfully, you're wrong. In fact, it's impossible for you to do something that you don't believe. The problem is the unconscious beliefs that we aren't even aware of. We're talking about a conscious belief versus an unconscious belief. While we will discuss this in detail in Secret #7, let me conclude this thought right now by stating that we can believe a hundred different things on different levels about the same issue. Sounds like we're all schizophrenic, right?

Fortunately, for most of us it doesn't get to that point. Suffice it to say, believing the truth in love and living that consciously and unconsciously in harmony, is an absolute caterpillar-to-butterfly transformation. This transformation is available to you right now through the secrets of this book. The incredible news of what we're offering you is a way to take flight that's not based on your effort or on being "right." There is a system in your body that can largely accomplish this automatically.

The only way I know to heal this problem permanently, completely, and totally, is to heal those cellular memories that are causing the problems that are being protected by the unconscious mind.

We're back again to asking how in the world you find those memories and, if you find them, how do you heal them? If talk therapy doesn't work … if behavioral modifications is just allowing you to cope and may actually be creating more stress, what we need is to remove the stress in order to heal. We have to get to the place where we can live what we believe is the truth, logically and rationally. God gave us the ability to reason logically and rationally so we could use it. To use it, we have to be able to heal the unconscious mind, what I call the "heart," and then live by that healed heart.

So, on to Secret #7 and more about the heart.

CHAPTER SEVEN

Secret #7:
When the Heart and the Head
Conflict, the Winner Is …

For years, as I have traveled around lecturing on psychology, spirituality, and natural healing, there's a little experiment I've done. Other people know about this test; in fact, my good friend Larry Napier told me about this test, and he did it all over the country as he lectured and had similar results.

It's very simple and you can see an illustration of it below. I draw a circle on a piece of paper and evenly divide the circle into four pie pieces. I number them "1," "2," "3," and "4." I also have a normal car or house key tied to the end of a string. I ask for a volunteer and have the person hold the string between their index and middle finger so that the key dangles over the center of the pie, right in the center of 1, 2, 3, and 4, about an inch or two above the paper.

The first instruction I give the person is to keep the key totally still and in the center of the pie between 1, 2, 3, and 4. If you are reading this, go ahead and see if you can do that. Most people do pretty well. Some people might be nervous, so their hands might be shaking a little bit or some people might have a health condition that causes the key to move a little bit, but most people can keep the key either right in the middle or very close to the middle.

In demonstrations we congratulate the person, and then I give them a second instruction. But before the second instruction, I remind them that instruction number one is still totally in place. Even with instruction number two, I tell them to keep that key right in the middle of the pie.

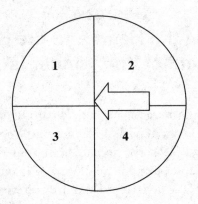

Now for instruction number two. As they hold the key still over the center, I tell them to imagine the key moving from pie piece number one to pie piece number two: "Back and forth between number one and number two. Just imagine it swinging between pie piece number one and piece number two. But remember command number one! Don't move it! Just imagine it moving."

What do you think happens? The results are really amazing. About 75 or 80 percent of the time, the key will start to move between pie piece number one and pie piece number two, usually very dramatically so that no one in the room would have any doubt about what is happening. It isn't just that it is moving around some and "maybe that could have been between one and two." It is obvious.

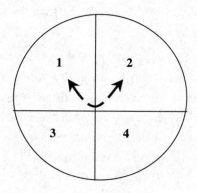

Then, I give the person a third command. Number one is still in place: Don't move the key. Number two is still in place. Now I tell them to imagine the key moving from two to four, two to four, two to four. But number one is still in place—don't move it. Again, 75-80 percent of the time, what will happen is the key will adjust. Sometimes it will go in a circle for just a second, and then it settles in and goes between two and four, two and four, two and four. The whole room will be amazed and clap.

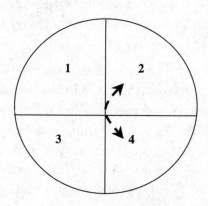

When we ask the person: "Did you try to do that?" Their response every time is "No!" They usually laugh and say, "I tried not to do it, I don't get it!"

Here's why this happens. I give the person two commands: I give them a head command and a heart command. I'm defining head as the conscious mind and heart as the unconscious mind, among other things. So the first command I give the person is a head command: "Do not move the key. Consciously focus on not moving the key." The second one is a heart command: "Imagine it moving." The imagination is a function of the unconscious and subconscious mind, even though we can manipulate it consciously. So I gave them both a head command and a heart command. *The heart command overrides the head command.*

THE HEART ALWAYS WINS

This is not a trauma situation like the instances we've been talking about up to this point. This is a no-danger, innocent, almost party-like situation. Still, the heart command overrides the head, and the key moves in the directions the unconscious is directing it to move. Pictures, not words, are the language of the heart, and the imagination is the picture maker. The image of the key moving is the heart command that overrides the head and causes the key to move.

How does that happen? When the person imagines the key moving, neurons start to fire in the brain. The brain sends energy frequencies and impulses down through the neck, then the shoulder, the arm, the hand, and finally the fingers. This causes the part of the fingers around the string to move, often so imperceptibly that no one can tell that they're moving anything, but it's exactly the movement that's needed to move the string and key on command. Sometimes we would even get creative and say, "I want you to imagine moving it in a circle," and it would. So when the heart and the head conflict, the heart always wins.

This is a critical point. We've talked about how Tracey and I consciously were on the same page and believed the same stuff and were so prepared for marriage. The woman who was raped consciously believed the right things; she was a Christian and believed that she should forgive the guy and tried to many, many times. She believed that she was clean before God and was not dirty or guilty or worthless. The problem was, she never *felt* that. She never experienced that. What she experienced was the opposite. The woman with the popsicle story consciously knew, "I've got an IQ of 180, I can do this better than all these people who are ahead of me, this is what I want in my life, and I can't think of any reason why Mom and I should have all this tension between us all the time."

But when the head and heart conflict, the heart wins. With Tracey and me, the unconscious pain memories started playing out in our marriage, so we blamed it on our current circumstances, but that's not what was going on. My client who was raped had subconscious and unconscious memories that were always there. She couldn't get rid of them. Insecurity, worthlessness, and anger would override her conscious mind and keep her from living the life she wanted to live. That's the way it always works when we have a very strong unconscious or subconscious belief that's based on a stimulus/ response pain memory. When this happens, the unconscious pain memory will win.

What does "win" mean? It means that we think, feel, and do things that we don't consciously want to do. It also means that the body's stress response is initiated when it shouldn't be. That's why it's so important to heal the memories that are the cause of this process.

THE SOURCE OF ALL ISSUES

Now, what happened with the 20-25 percent of people where the key and string did not move? It appears the heart did not override the head. Whenever that happened, I would ask the person, "When I told you to imagine the key and string moving, were you able to do that? Were you able in your mind's eye to see it moving?" I've never had one situation where the person said they were able to see it. Not one.

What does that mean? It means, first of all, that they were not able to activate the mechanisms in the heart that would cause the heart to override. Secondly, and this is a bigger concern, people who cannot imagine, who have lost that ability, usually have more unconscious and subconscious pain memories than any other group of people. As a protection their minds have shut down their ability to imagine, because everything they see activates images that hurt (remember, those memories are encoded and recalled in the form of images). Their unconscious minds shut down that capacity so they can try to live a halfway normal life. However, it's still working all the time. Even though in their current circumstances they can't see their memories and use their imaginations in that way, they still feel the pain and think the destructive, painful thoughts about themselves, others, and circumstances, and still do things that are not the things they want to do.

There is a verse in the Bible: "Guard your heart above everything else because from it flow the issues of life" (Proverbs 4:23). I am told by a scholar that if you go to the original text of that passage and ask the question, "What percentage of the issues of life?"—the answer would be 100 percent. So according to the Bible, which I believe is non-negotiable truth (you are free to have your own opinion), if you have an issue in your life, the origin of it is a heart issue. If you don't heal the heart issue, you may knock back the symptoms some, but you cannot have permanent, complete healing of the issue, because you have not healed the source.[14]

So this is Secret #7: *When the head and heart conflict, the heart wins.* We know that these signals sent from the heart—the cellular memories of the heart—activate the stress response in the body, which leads to all of our problems.

UNCONSCIOUS AND CONSCIOUS INTENTION

I had the pleasure of spending a day with Professor William Tiller from Stanford. Dr. Tiller has published many books, was one of the stars of the movie, *What the Bleep do We Know?* and is considered by many to be one of the prominent quantum physicists of our day. Several golden nuggets came out of my conversations that day with professor Tiller. Here are two of them:

1. There is an unconscious intention for most issues in life. Everyone is talking about the conscious intention—which is real and important, but not the whole story.

---

14 As a side note, we ourselves are committed to following Jesus. Therefore we believe that the deepest healing comes through Jesus Christ. That is the faith we believe and that is what we live. In fact, I believe my faith was a vital element in my discovering The Healing Codes, as I described in the Preface to this book. (For more specifics on our beliefs and philosophy, turn to "A Word about Us and Our Philosophy" at the end of the book.) But we're not trying to force that on anyone who is reading this. The Healing Code works, in our experience, no matter what you believe, no matter what age you are, no matter what sex you are, no matter what nationality or ethnicity you are. Double-A batteries work in whatever device is made to work from that power source. The Healing Code works because it operates according to the hard and fast laws of nature called quantum physics. They are based on the way the universe was created.

2. When the unconscious intention and conscious intention conflict, the unconscious wins.

Dr. Bruce Lipton says much the same thing. In a program Ben and I did with him, Dr. Lipton stated that it's almost impossible to change our issues through willpower because the subconscious mind is more than a million times more powerful than our willpower. He also said that you almost have to have something like The Healing Codes to change those issues.

HEART ISSUES ARE SPIRITUAL ISSUES

I'm going to make some bold statements here.

In Secret #1 we said that every time we have a health problem or relationship problem we should ask, "What is the stress that is causing this?" I believe we should go farther and, whenever we have a health problem, a relationship problem, a problem with our career, we should ask, "What is the heart problem I have that is the source of this, and how do I heal it?" You may be thinking, *Okay. Now we are getting into the area of spirituality*, and my response would be, "You are absolutely right."

The Healing Code, though it is a physical mechanism in the body that you physically turn on and activate, is also a spiritual exercise in that it heals heart issues. Does it forgive people for you? Does it take away sin from your life? Absolutely not. Those things only you and God can do.

What The Healing Code does is heal the destructive energy pattern of the memory that contains a wrong belief that is making you afraid when you should not be afraid and activating your body's stress response system when it should not be activated, leading to health issues and every other problem we know of. I believe what we see here is the Bible and science coming together in perfect unity, but the Bible said it much, much earlier: "From the heart flow all the issues of life."

Now for some bold statements based on what we've been talking about. My spiritual mentor, Larry Napier, taught me most of these life-changing truths some twenty years ago, before they had been proven by science. The more I learn and experience, the more I realize they are true. They changed my life then, now, and forever. I thank Larry for loving me, and I share these with you now in love. I hope they will have a similar impact in your life. Here they are:

> **You are who you are in your heart.** You may tell people, "This is who I am, this is what I believe, this is what I've done, this is what I'm going to do," but who you really are is who you are in your heart, because when the head and heart conflict, the heart wins.

> **What you really believe is what you believe in your heart**. The story of how Tracey and I agreed on all of our conscious beliefs but less than a year later we both wanted a divorce shows how our unconscious beliefs are what we end up living by most of the time. What you really believe is what you believe in your heart.

> **You are where you are based on what's in your heart**. The stimulus/response belief system, when it is activated, will take you back to whatever age you were when that pain memory was created. The Wall Street woman when she was thirty-something years old in her high-rise office in Manhattan was five years old many, many times a day, whenever that popsicle memory was reactivated. And she felt like a five-year-old. She felt helpless, she felt angry, she felt worthless, she felt like "I can't do this job," even though if anything she

was overqualified, and she and everyone else knew that consciously. But that's not the reality of what she was living. You are now where you were then anytime one of those pain memories is reactivated. You will revert to where you were when that pain event occurred, and the age that it occurred, with the reasoning ability of that age, and the feelings and emotions.

You do what you do based on what's in your heart. Consciously, we can make all these wonderful plans. We can even have the ability to carry them out. But if we have pain memories about those same actions and those same issues, we will end up responding to those pain memories whether we want to or not and acting on the beliefs of the pain memories until we can heal them. When we are not doing what we want to do, or at least are not doing it as consistently as we need to, to accomplish what we want in our lives, that is evidence that these heart-pain memories are being reactivated and are causing us to do something that we don't want. This includes unwanted thoughts and feelings as well.

The heart is programmed to protect. It is the number one job of the heart to protect you from having painful, possibly fatal things from happening and especially from happening again. That is why when the head and heart conflict the heart wins, because the heart is programmed to protect. It does this by stimulating the body's stress response. If the stress response kicks in when it shouldn't kick in, it causes us to be afraid when we should not be afraid. If the head and heart conflict and the heart wins in a destructive way that affects our health or career or relationships, or keeps us from being at peace, it is because of fear in our hearts. We may not consciously feel the fear, but that is what's being resonated to our cells.

Your priorities are determined by what's in your heart. If you ask a hundred people how they go about prioritizing things in their lives, it's very likely that all one hundred would respond that they decide what's important and what to do first based on a rational, logical examination of their facts and circumstances. However, how you actually prioritize is determined by what you value, and what you value is based on what's in your heart. Does that mean we're just robots and a rational, logical look at life is meaningless? Of course not! It is a factor in the process, and as long as the heart agrees with our rational thinking, there's no problem. However, when our cellular memory dictates a fear-based belief, it will literally cause us to examine the same rational fact but come to a not necessarily logical or congruent conclusion.

THE HEART RULES

When he was twelve, my son, Harry, watched the original *Jaws* movie. (My wife and I are still debating whether that was a good idea.) Harry has loved the water from the time he was an infant. One time when Harry was about two years old, we were walking on the grounds of a hotel in the middle of winter. To our amazement, Harry jumped into the swimming pool. This happened more than once at different times and in different places. Harry swims like a fish—doesn't matter whether it's a pool, lake, or ocean. He loves it. After watching *Jaws*, I asked Harry if he wanted to go to the lake. You could see deep consideration in his eyes and face as if he were examining the possibilities as a thirty-five year old would examine his taxes. After about a minute, Harry declined and said that he would prefer to stay home and play with Legos.

When I questioned Harry about whether his decision had anything to do with the *Jaws* movie, Harry responded, "Absolutely not." He was just really excited about designing some Legos buildings. And he was fairly convincing in his argument. I asked Harry if it would be okay to test him and see if he had a cellular fear memory from the movie. Sure enough, he did have a destructive cellular memory. Harry did a Healing Code, which took about 4 minutes, and guess what? Over that 4 minutes, Harry's priorities totally changed! His rational, logical thinking totally changed. Now, Harry decided he could do Legos anytime and would absolutely love to go to the lake—"How soon can we go?"

This doesn't happen only to twelve year olds. It happens to all of us constantly. What we think are rational, logical decisions based on the truth are oftentimes an unconscious rationalization of values and priorities that are based on destructive heart memories.

This process is almost always unconscious, at least until you start to look around and find some of these memories or heal some of these memories. Sometimes they become conscious once they've been healed because the heart doesn't feel like it has to protect them anymore, but usually these things are unconscious. So I yell at my wife and I think, "Why did I do that?" I eat when I don't want to. I don't make the calls that I need to make in order to be successful in my work. I keep making excuses and telling myself day after day I'm going to do it. I may even start lying to my wife or to my employer and all I know is I can't seem to do it. It's because I have pain memories in my heart that are being reactivated and they need to be healed.

So the only way to live and love from the heart in the way we want to is to heal the destructive memories of the heart.

THE HEART-BODY CONNECTION

Let me make one more statement. We've been talking in these last four Secrets about things that we would call non-physical: memories, beliefs, actions, thoughts. However, please don't forget the first Secret, which is that these memories, these beliefs, these heart issues control the physiology of our body. These wrong beliefs kick the body's stress response into action when it should not be kicked in. When that happens it causes, over time, almost all illness and disease that we know of. It shuts off our cells, causes the immune system to be turned off, and we end up with every kind of health problem we can imagine. Both the physical problems and the non-physical problems all originate from these heart issues, from these cellular memories that create destructive energy frequencies that send our body into the stress response when it should not.

So there we have it: Secrets #1 through 7. We believe that this material has never been put together in this way before. Some of it is new insight and new research as to how the body, mind and heart work. We believe that for the first time you can take all of this information and all of this truth and heal your heart issues, heal your cellular memories, and remove the stress from your life so that you can do the things you have dreamed of all your life in achievement, relationships, career, peak performance, preventative health, healing a health problem, and your relationships with your family members. Anything in your life, we believe, can be greatly enhanced by understanding how all of this works and then using The Healing Code to heal the source of all of your problems—your heart issues and the destructive, painful cellular memories of your heart that contain wrong beliefs.

Welcome to a new life.

The conclusion of the matter, based on all seven Secrets, is two truths:

1. **To heal your problems you have to heal the stress**. There's just no other way. It's the one thing everybody agrees on, including the federal government, traditional health, alternative health, research going back twenty years, and twenty million web sites. There's just no way around it; you have to heal the stress if you want permanent, long-term, complete healing for your problems.

2. **To heal the stress you have to heal your memories.** According to research from Southwestern University Medical School and Stanford University Medical School, the thing that causes the stress response in the body is not just our current circumstances. It is our wrong beliefs, our destructive cellular memories that are encoded and stored in our hearts, in our minds—what the Bible calls the heart.

IS WHAT YOU'RE CURRENTLY DOING WORKING?

After those two conclusions, here's the question: *Are you acting on them?* Whatever you're doing right now to try to succeed or to heal or to resolve or to cope—whatever word you want to use—are you accomplishing these two things? Are you healing the stress? Are you healing the cellular memories that are causing the stress? If you're not, the chances of your healing your problem totally, completely, and permanently are very, very slim.

Why is that? If you're not doing these two things, you're trying to fix your problems by working on symptoms of the problem. In other words, you're trying to get the pain to go away, but you're not dealing with the source of the pain.

Suppose you have a pain in your abdomen that keeps recurring over and over and over again, and you constantly have to take Advil or Tylenol to knock out the pain. You have this gut feeling that "You know, this shouldn't be happening," and a fear, "I wonder if this is cancer or a gallbladder problem or an intestinal problem or an ulcer or something like that." But instead of dealing with that and finding out what the problem is and healing it, you just keep taking Tylenol and Advil to knock out the pain.

We all recognize you're not going to heal that problem by just knocking out the pain, and neither are you going to heal the problems of your life by just trying to cope or to manage or to think about it differently with a more positive attitude. You have to heal the source. That is what The Healing Code is all about.

WIDE-RANGING EFFECTS

We believe The Healing Codes® are what has been predicted by the greatest minds of our time as the future of medicine. Only, its scope encompasses more than medicine. It heals relationship problems, mental health issues, career problems, peak performance issues—you name it—because it all has the same source, which is stress caused by destructive, painful cellular memories in our unconscious minds.

Recently, we gave a seminar in a major city in the Midwest. The first person who came up to me that evening was a gentleman who had started doing The Healing Codes seven months before. His problem was not feelings or beliefs or negative thinking, at least not consciously. His problem was congestive heart failure, high blood pressure, his heart muscle only using 20 percent contraction, edema, and a number of other related physical problems. He did The Healing Codes for seven months and basically didn't think they had done him any good at all. The day before our seminar he had gone back for his yearly checkup with his cardiologist. After running exhaustive tests, the doctor came into the room scratching his head and said to this gentleman, "Whatever you're doing, don't stop." His blood pressure was completely normal, the edema was gone, and the contraction of the heart muscle was up to 50 percent. They removed medication and told him that these results were basically impossible.

We have hundreds of pages of these stories. Some are mentioned in this book, but feel free to check some of them out on our website (www.thehealingcodebook.com). Many of the tests that were performed on my friend above scan for energy frequency, as we talked about earlier. When those frequencies change, the results of the tests change. When the results of the test change, doctors end up scratching their heads and saying, "This is impossible," and, "Whatever you're doing, don't stop." All of this healing in the body is the result of healing an energy problem. When the confusion, negative emotions, and destructive thinking patterns related to a particular issue heal, then the person is able to see the truth, and the frequency of their cells comes back into balance and health.

Now you have all seven Secrets. I hope you now understand why you have the problems you have and that you also have hope like never before that you can be healed. But let's not leave anything to chance. Let's go now to putting all of the secrets together in the form of five steps to getting the results that you want in your life.

CHAPTER EIGHT

It's All about Results

In the movie *Jerry McGuire*, Tom Cruise starred as a sports agent who hit a professional mid-life crisis. The pop-culture take away line from that movie was from a memorable scene with his co-star, Cuba Gooding, Jr. Gooding played a wide-receiver for a professional sports team. He's trying to get a contract he felt he deserved but that he'd never really lived up to. In an intense moment of truth for Cruise, Gooding shared his mantra as a professional athlete, which was, "Show me the money!" In other words, talk is cheap; I want results! This is precisely where this book started. I made a promise to you that I would "show you the money" as far as your health, life, and prosperity are concerned. In other words, "How can you get the results you want in your life?"

Before we pull all our loose ends together, an interesting side note is that Cruise's character in that movie ended up telling his professional athlete client that he would show him the money when he started playing from the heart instead of his head. Fairy tales come true in the movies all the time, and this one was no exception. Gooding learned to play from his heart, and Cruise was able to "show him the money" because of that.

This is a pretty good encapsulation of this entire book. If you learn to live from your heart, you will get the results you seek in your life.

We hope you see by now that your problems come from the heart, as do the solutions. How do you put all of this together in a practical way so that this is not just theory that sounds good and makes sense but doesn't create any lasting change in your life? Try this little exercise from Walt Disney.

Walt Disney was a genius in anybody's book. He was a genius in many areas: animation, drawing, business and others. But maybe the biggest area of greatness for him was imagination. Disney developed a process in his company called "storyboarding" that is now used all over the world in corporate America, churches, small businesses, movies, the arts, you name it. Storyboarding is a process that organizes imagination and then makes it practically useable. The way I was taught storyboarding started with turning your imagination loose and writing down anything and everything that comes to mind as a possibility for whatever topic you're brainstorming. That's where I want you to start. Let your mind go free. Let your spirit soar about what your life can be from now on.

Now, write down right here what you desire, need, seek, want, require, etc. Be as specific as possible without any limitations. See it, feel it, taste it, touch it, smell it, experience it. Brainstorm.

_____

_____

_____

_____

RESULTS

Let me throw a monkey wrench in and impose two limitations. These are truth and love. Now look at everything you came up with and see if it will fit in the container of truth and love. If it won't, mark it off.

This can vary from person to person. For instance, Bill Gates, before he became the Bill Gates that we all know, started as a normal person, not a billionaire. I haven't had the pleasure of asking him this question, but maybe when he brainstormed, he saw being a billionaire, so for him, that dream of his imagination would be in the context of truth and love. However, I have a feeling that if I could go back in time and ask Mother Teresa when she was a young nun if one of the results that she wanted was to personally be a billionaire, she would have said, "No way. That's not my mission. I'm not called to that." For her, being a billionaire would not have been in the context of truth and love.

I know you may be thinking, "How do I know what the truthful and loving result is for me?" You're not going to like my answer, but it's the only one I can give you and be truthful. You will know. You may not know in a day or a week or six months. But if you keep seeking the truth in love, you will find the answer to those questions. As you clean out the destructive memories of your heart, that vision will become clear for you. Remember that it is our destructive cellular memories that cause us to believe something that's not true, that make us afraid when we should not be afraid, and that activate the stress response of the body. So as you heal those cellular memories, you will find a clarity of purpose that you have never experienced before.

This is a life-long journey, but many of these things you already know. For instance, the results that I want in my own life are: I want to be the best husband that I can be; I desire to be the most loving father that I am capable of for Harry and George; I want each and every client I work with to walk away not only with health, but feeling truly cared about. These are the most important results in my life and they are no-brainers. I heard it said in a seminar once that no matter what people say they want in life, when probing questions continued to be asked, what everyone wants is the same: love, joy, and peace. I confirmed it through straw polls with my own clients, asking them what they want and then probing deeper and deeper until we get to the core of what they really want. And it comes down to those three things. Of course, many people never realize that that's what they really want, which is an entirely different matter and a heart issue in and of itself.

THE POWER OF BELIEFS

To get results, you have to have power. Just like a vacuum cleaner is useless until you plug it in, or an automobile without gasoline won't run, or a person without food can't function properly, there has to be power before any results are achieved. The greater the power, the greater the results.

Many years ago, the U.S. ended a great war by dropping two atomic bombs on Japan. It ended the war because there was no other weapon in the world that could release the power of an atomic bomb. It was a quantum breakthrough in weaponry and anyone who didn't have it couldn't compete. The Japanese knew this, and rather than suffer annihilation, they surrendered. Up until this time, there were other countries trying to develop and/or steal the secret of atomic power, but the United States got there first.

One of the fascinating things about the discovery of atomic technology is that at its essence, power is not created, it is released. In other words, the power that leveled two cities in 1945 was right there and available in particles called atoms the whole time. The secret was in finding a way to pull the atoms apart and release the power from within. Of course, that release of power was tremendously destructive. Nuclear power plants use the same power for more constructive purposes. Power is available for any purpose; the point is it is available to be harnessed. Since the destructive use of atomic power, we have discovered how to use it for good purposes— to power homes and even some vehicles.

Tremendous power is inside you today in the "issues of the heart" and it can be constructive or destructive. It can block your goals, relationships and create illness and disease. Or it can empower you to fantastic accomplishments, wonderful relationships, and tremendous health. You have all the tools and resources you need to achieve the results that you wrote down above. You just need to release that power.

How do you do that? *Power is released by belief.*

We can see this power of belief in what is known in medicine as the placebo effect, where someone is given a sugar pill but told that it's a new miracle drug to solve whatever their problem is. The amazing thing is that many people will actually experience the desired result without taking anything that could seemingly achieve that result. In other words, the problem goes away with the sugar pill! In fact, in a nationwide survey of American doctors that was reported in 2008, half of all doctors admitted that they prescribed placebos. Surveys in Denmark, Israel, Britain, Sweden and New Zealand have found similar results.[15] Ethics aside, why do doctors prescribe sugar pills? Because placebos work!

There is more proof of the power of belief: the flip side of the placebo affect, called "the nocebo effect." Doctors know about this, too: what happens when people are given a placebo and warned of the negative effects it may have. They experience those negative effects! "In double-blind clinical trials of antidepressants, even those participants receiving a sugar pill report side effects like gastrointestinal discomfort if investigators have warned them at the outset that those effects are likely," reports *Time* magazine on a famous Pain study led by Italian neuroscientist Martina Amanzio.[16]

Furthermore, the patients receiving placebos developed symptoms similar to the side effects of the drugs they thought

---

15 "Half of Doctors Routinely Prescribe Placebos," *The New York Times*, October 23, 2008 (http://www.nytimes.com/2008/10/24/health/24placebo.html?ref=health).

16 "The Flip Side of Placebos: The Nocebo Effect," John Cloud, *Time*, October 13, 2009 (http://www.time.com/time/health/article/0,8599,1929869,00.html?iid=sphere-inline-sidebar).

they were taking. "Patients who took sugar pills tended to report nocebo problems consistent with whatever drug they thought they might have swallowed. No one who thought they could be taking an NSAID or triptan reported memory problems or tingling, but some who thought they might have taken anticonvulsants did. Likewise, only placebo groups in the NSAID trials reported side effects like stomach upset and dry mouth."

I was told of a study recently where they had given subjects who were all in chronic pain a placebo and told them that it was some spectacular new form of morphine that could relieve their pain like a miracle. Sure enough, many of the subjects' pain went away. This has happened many thousands of times before in research all over the world. The thing I'd never heard of before was the next thing they did in this particular study. They went inside the body to see what had actually happened in the people who had taken the placebo that caused the people's pain to go away. What they discovered was simply amazing. The body had literally produced an extremely high grade of the natural equivalent of morphine, and that's why the pain went away. How did this happen? No one knows. What we do know is that placebo studies going back more than fifty years prove beyond the shadow of a doubt that the body and the mind are capable of doing things that we would believe to be impossible. What causes these remarkable results? The person believes it. I don't think I could come up with any better examples of how believing releases the power for our results than the "nocebo effect."

Let me go one other place with this. Results don't happen only with sugar pills and body chemistry. Results also happen with our thinking, feeling and actions. Remember the story of the young Chinese karate student from the "I Believe" Secret? The young student who broke those bricks that no master in history had done before was experiencing the opposite of the placebo effect. Placebo is a little power being released because you believe, but you are believing a lie and the results are not sustained. The young karate student believed the whole truth—100 percent of the truth without 1 percent of doubt, fear, or confusion. Because of that belief, miraculous, and some would say impossible, results occurred. That is the difference between living your life based on destructive cellular memories that contain lies versus living your life believing the truth.

THE SURPRISING TRUTH ABOUT "AFFIRMATIONS"

I have to stop for a moment here to address the topic of affirmations. For several decades now, and big time for the last twenty years, the self-help world has been booming with affirmations. Many "gurus" have become wealthy by teaching people that all they have to do to get anything they want is to believe, and the right affirmation will create the belief and "magically" bring them the new car, millions of dollars, the love of their life, or even physical healing.

The problem is that this almost never works. Good people spend thousands of dollars and decades of their lives on this "placebo"-based practice and wind up in a vicious cycle that leaves them disillusioned, poorer, and often out of time.

For about two years I tested these types of "name it and claim it" affirmations. I hooked people up to HRV (the medical test for stress) and had them say affirmations such as, "My new car is on the way to me," or, "My cancer is healing right now."

Guess what? Almost every time, their HRV crashed—meaning massive new stress from saying that affirmation. And remember, stress is the cause of just about everything bad that we know of. I was so thrilled when a new study from the University of Waterloo in Canada in 2009 tested affirmations. This was headline news all over the world. The results were that for the vast majority of people, these types of affirmations not only don't work, they make things *worse*.

That's why for many years, I have advocated what I call "truth focus statements." Yes, they are positive, but they are things that you actually believe. So instead of "my cancer is healing," when you really don't believe it is, the truth focus statement might be, "I want my cancer to heal, believe it can, and ask God to help me with that." When people say a truth focus statement while hooked up to HRV, their stress tends to decrease. What's the difference? It's the same difference between a placebo and the real thing. One statement you believe, and it's positive. The other statement you don't believe—so to your heart you are telling a lie.

BELIEF AND BEHAVIOR

We always do what we believe, and everything we do, we do because of something we believe. If you're doing something that you don't want to be doing, it's because you have a wrong belief. To change the unwanted behavior, you have to change the belief. The placebo effect seems to illustrate that very nicely, but I'm sorry to say there's one problem. Another universal truth about the placebo effect is that the desired result is almost never sustained. What that means is that you will get a "flash in the pan" taste of the result that you want in your life or your health, but it won't last. Because of that, the placebo effect can actually be very dangerous. There are hundreds of millions of dollars spent every year because something sounds good. When people try it they think they experience some benefit, but permanent change does not occur. However, because they felt some benefit from whatever the pill or program was, they may try month after month, year after year to make something happen in their lives without the power to actually make it happen.

Why are placebo results not sustained? If you think about it, it's simple: because the people aren't believing the truth. They're believing that a sugar pill is a miracle drug. However, even though they believe it, it's still not true. In order for results to be sustained, there has to be *sustained* power.

You can't just plug the vacuum cleaner into the outlet for thirty seconds and get your rug cleaned. You have to keep it plugged in. Sustained power only occurs through believing the whole truth. It's a surprising point that believing literally anything will release some power. As crazy as it seems, even a lie will release some power. That is what makes this phenomenon extremely dangerous. It is easy, especially when we are sick or needy in some way, to be seduced by a little power or a taste of the result that we so long for. We grab hold of it and are pulled into a dark pit. The lie now has us. How do you get out of the pit? By discarding the lie and embracing the truth, the whole truth, and nothing but the truth. That's not as easy as it sounds, because when you are embracing the lie, you will tend to be confused. More on confusion below.

BELIEVE THE TRUTH, CHANGE REALITY

An interesting thing about quantum physics (atomic power is intertwined with quantum physics) is that in quantum physics, reality is changed by the way you look at it. In other words, you literally change the physical makeup of the particles and physical reality by the angle at which you look or observe tiny particles. The angle at which you look at anything is determined by what you believe. As we've been saying through this whole book, if you can get to the place where you're looking at your own life in truth and love, it will absolutely change your reality and results.

So believing the truth in love about your life will release power that will produce results ... the best results ... the very best results. We're talking health, prosperity, intimate relationships, fulfillment, and of course, love, joy, and peace. Now which results will you get? Only you and God can answer that question. See, I don't know if you're Bill Gates or Mother Teresa. Maybe you don't know. But if you clean out your heart junk, you will know your mission, your destiny.

So how do you believe the truth in love? It all begins with actual ... TRUTH. But sometimes you have to cut through the forest of lies to get to it.

HOW CONFUSION BLOCKS TRUTH

Step number one should be to heal your destructive heart memories. Why? Because they cause you to believe something that's not true. What is that called? Confusion. What is the result of confusion? Taking the wrong road. Believing the truth gives us the feeling that "I know this is right!" but when we believe something that's not the truth, we are confused and we don't know which direction to take.

Confusion is caused by three things. Number one is cellular memories that conflict with each other. In other words, you have voices from the past telling you what to do, but the voices are telling you to do different things at the same time. Number two is conflict between the conscious and unconscious mind (what we call the head and the heart—see Secret #7, When the Head and the Heart Conflict). Number three cause of confusion is you're being "dumbed down" because of stress (see Secret #1). Stress turns our rational reasoning down or off. Since about 90 percent of us are walking around in some degree of physiological stress, our ability to think correctly and clearly is diminished to the degree that we are in stress.

Are you in confusion right now? If so, which of the three causes are you experiencing? Many people have all three operating at once.

In our home, we have a huge enclosed bookcase that my parents had shipped from Hong Kong piece by piece. It takes up a whole wall in our living room. People who come to visit us frequently know my background in psychology, so they look at all the books on my bookshelves and say, "Wow, you've read a ton of books!" I have to be honest and tell them that I probably haven't read three books in that bookcase. Tracey read all of those books and many more over the twelve years she was desperately looking for relief from depression. I don't know how many times over those years I would see Tracey reading a book or listening to a book on tape or hearing a lecture and I would become so excited thinking that maybe this would be the thing that would bring the truth to Tracey's heart and break through the bondage of her depression.

What would happen, and it must have happened five hundred times over those years, is that I would ask Tracey how her book was or if she was learning anything. Her response was identical every single time. Four words: "I don't get it."

Many times I would ask for clarification. Do you mean you don't understand it? Tracey would respond back: "Of course I understand it. I've read the same paragraph four times—I can quote it. I just don't get it. It doesn't make any difference in my life." This from a woman with a 129 IQ! This was one of the great mysteries of the first twelve years of our marriage for me, because many of those things Tracey was exposing her mind to were wonderful, fabulous truths. She was reading the words of wisdom of many of the greatest minds of our time, as well as timeless wisdom from the Bible, Mother Teresa, and more. How could she not understand this? How could this not make any difference? How could this not apply to her life? It all applied to her life! Why couldn't she see that?

Once I learned the truths that are in this book you now hold, I understood. The answer was that she couldn't see the truth. She was in such a state of confusion because of all the untruths and lies in her heart (and remember when the head and heart conflict, the heart wins) that she couldn't understand the truth. Now did she have truthful beliefs in her heart, too? Absolutely! Lots of them. But that's exactly what happens when you have both truths and lies (which on some level you believe) that conflict in your heart. Both seem right at a certain level. It causes confusion. We may feel better about one alternative than another, but we still have confusion and are not sure.

THE PEACE TEST

What is the litmus test for this confusion? It is peace, or an absence of peace. If I have peace about a certain belief or course of action, that is the indicator that I am believing the truth in love. If I have anxiety, sadness, confusion, second thoughts, a nagging feeling in my chest or the pit of my stomach, then I've got something in my heart that I'm believing that is interfering with my ability to believe the whole, real truth. In other words, I'm not believing the truth in love and I will not get the results I want.

I need to say one more word about this peace we've been speaking of. Many people confuse peace with two other things. One is a sense of happiness and contentment because "things are going my way." This is not peace. It's fortunate circumstances. How do you know which one you're dealing with? Do you have that peace even if the circumstances turn against you, or do you plummet into confusion, depression, and anxiety? True peace is not dependent on circumstances.

The second thing people confuse with peace is feeling numb. "I don't feel confusion, I don't feel anxiety, I don't feel fear, I don't feel pain ... I don't feel anything!" This is not peace, either. It is usually evidence of massive destructive cellular memories, so massive that your heart has turned off your "feeler" so that you can survive because everything you were feeling was causing so much pain.

THE POWER OF FULL TRUTH

To get the results that I promised at the beginning of the book, you need to believe the truth.

When I was a young child, I went to see a movie that absolutely enchanted me. It was one of the best movies I'd ever seen at that time in my life. I promptly came home and jumped off our roof with an umbrella. No, I was not trying to commit suicide; I'd just seen *Mary Poppins*. Obviously, after watching Julie Andrews flying through the air with her umbrella, I believed I could, too. You want evidence that I believed it? I jumped off the roof! Everything we do is because of something we believe. It would have been impossible for me to jump off the roof if I didn't believe that I'd be okay. I honestly and truthfully believed that I could fly with that umbrella, but that did not get me the results of flying through the air that I wanted. The only way to get the results is to believe the truth.

You say, "Wait a minute, I thought that power is released when you believe anything, even something that's not true. So where's the power in the jumping-off-the-roof story?" Number one, in my heart. At the moment I jumped off that roof, I felt like Superman—and I hadn't taken any pills. I was strong, I was free, I was exhilarated ... that's power! Number two, I jumped. If you lined one hundred kids who were my age on that rooftop and asked them to jump, how many do you think would actually jump? Probably none! Even if you got out your wallet or candy or videos and tried to bribe them, they still probably wouldn't jump. My point is that it takes enormous power to get a little kid to go against every ounce of survival instinct in order to do something that's in his heart to do. That is power, and that is results. The problem is, I didn't get the results that I wanted and, of course, the results were not sustained.

So I had a piece of truth, which was I went to this movie and saw someone else flying with umbrellas, but missed the part that flying off the roof defies the hard and fast law of nature called gravity. If instead of coming home from the theater and immediately jumping, I'd gotten more information and known the truth, I'm convinced now that I wouldn't have jumped. How would that have happened? I would have looked up light and gravity and falling in our encyclopedia. I would certainly have asked for my parents' opinion, and if I was desperate enough, even my older brother. I may have gone to kindergarten the next day and asked the teacher if she had seen the movie and what she thought about jumping off the roof. You get the point. I would have had enough new, true information in my heart so that I wouldn't have that lie in my heart and the potential to hurt myself pretty badly.

THE MISSING INGREDIENT

You may have figured out by now that there's something missing. So let's do a little review. Number one is that we need to know the results that we want. Number two is that it takes power to achieve those results. Number three is that believing releases power. And number four is that we must believe the truth in order to get the sustained results that we desire. So what's missing? It's back to Tracey's four words. Do you remember them? "I don't get it." In other words, we can have all of the truth that we need to achieve our sustained results, but still not release any power. This was what was happening with Tracey until the spring of 2001. This is the biggest issue in this whole book. Most people have access to more truth than ever before, especially in this Internet age. That should mean more sustained results than ever before, but that's not what's happening. Yes, we are living as long as people have ever lived, and in many cases longer. However, we are getting sicker and sicker.

I had a call from a gentleman last night whose young child has struggled for years with asthma. He was relating to me how in his son's class there are so many other children who struggle with asthma, and it's not just his class, but every class in the whole school. You may not know it, but a number of years ago, asthma was pretty rare. Now it's commonplace. A number of years ago, ADD and ADHD were not terms that were ever heard. Today it's a major issue for every school in the world. In 1971 President Richard Nixon declared war on cancer. At that time, cancer was the 8th or 9th cause of death in America. As of 2009, cancer is the second leading cause of death in America (after heart disease). We're losing the war, and it's not just to physical illness. Mental illness has been on the rise for years. I heard from a woman recently that almost all of the women at her woman's Bible class are on either an antidepressant or antianxiety medication. Up until recently, Valium was the number one prescribed medication of all time. Relationships seem disposable in a way that would have been a community stigma a number of years ago.

How can this be happening when we're making so many medical advances? You should know by now—because those advances have nothing to do with the source of the problem. The source is destructive cellular memories. Society deluges all of us on a daily basis with negative images through television, movies, magazines, and newspapers, but we don't even realize it most of the time.

I saw an ad for a movie recently and the bullet points that are supposed to make you want to see the movie said: "Sex, Murder, Betrayal, Deception." Guess what? Those are the things that make up cellular memories that are blocking your results and making you sick. Seeing a good movie can infuse healing, healthy, and truthful memories in us, just as a bad one can harm us.

But back to what's missing. The key to believing the truth is UNDERSTANDING.

UNDERSTANDING AND THE WHOLE TRUTH

Remember the research by Dr. Bruce Lipton from Stanford University Medical School that 100 percent of the time the cause of the stress that makes us sick is a wrong belief. What is a wrong belief? It is believing something that's not true. It is actually more accurate to call it "a misunderstanding of the truth." In just about every destructive memory, there is some truth. The client of mine from Secret #5 who was raped had a lot of things about the memory of the rape that were truthful. In fact, the majority of what she remembered was truthful. The main thing that was not truthful was her interpretation of what the rape meant, in this case, "I am worthless; I am never safe; no one will ever look at me the same way." Somehow she looked at the fact and truth of what happened to her and came to a wrong conclusion. She misunderstood the truth. In the popsicle story, the great majority of what that sweet woman believed was true, too. Her mom did tell her she couldn't have a popsicle, her mom did give one to her sister. Her mom did tell her that if she had a good lunch she could have one too, but in spite of that she misinterpreted, misunderstood, and came to a wrong conclusion. Her conclusions were very similar to the woman who was raped: "I'm unlovable; I'm worthless; something's wrong with me." The lack of power and results in the two women's lives were similar, as well. They were much more intensified in the woman who was raped, yes, but there were very similar underlying beliefs.

In the three cases of Tracey with her depression, the woman who was raped, and the woman with the popsicle story, once they healed the lies of their hearts, they were able to understand the truth. They believed, and power was released, and all of them have had sustained results ever since.

At first glance, it may seem like a daunting task to have to find the whole truth about any issue before you can have sustained results with it. Don't despair; it's not that difficult. If we have a relatively clean heart, we will often know the truth in our heart the first time we see or hear it. It resonates and we feel it to the deepest core of who we are. That's because we have a mechanism inside us called the "conscience." Its sole purpose is to help us find these truths. However, when there are too many lies in the heart related to a given subject, the voice of the conscience is drowned out, or at least confused, by competing and disagreeing voices. The key is cleaning out the misunderstandings of the heart, which are imbedded in our cellular memories.

Until recently, this was anything but a simple proposition. People would spend years in counseling or therapy, and like Tracey, buy a library of self-help books, usually with little success. This is because we have been trying to heal these cellular memories with tools that are not capable of healing them. Since 2001, with the discovery of The Healing Codes, we now have a simple tool that will consistently and predictably heal the source rather than address symptoms. More on The Healing Codes in the next chapter.

THE PLACE OF PRAYER

I don't want to leave the impression that before The Healing Codes were discovered, issues of the heart could not be healed.

What heals the issues of the heart is replacing lies with the truth, and this is certainly at the heart of prayer and what the Bible teaches. The problem is, even few Christians really follow this process of allowing God to heal the heart junk through replacing the lies with truth. The Healing Code does not work on the level of prayer and is not a replacement for it. It is more on the level of and a replacement for the coping strategies mentioned earlier. The Healing Code, as we've shown, works much better because it heals the source, rather than attempting to alleviate symptoms or cope. The Healing Code works with prayer, as you will see in the next chapter. I always pray first about anything, asking God to work through whatever means he chooses—including The Healing Codes.

Now let's take a look at all five steps to get the results you want that I promised you in the first chapter of the book: Results, Power, Belief, Understanding, Truth. If you have the courage to apply these steps to the thing you want to change in your life, you will get the results that you seek.

Does that mean that whatever result you decide you want before you start the process is the exact result you will end up with? No, it doesn't. It means you will get the best result, perhaps one that you might not even be able to imagine now.

YOU BE THE JUDGE

Okay. Time for you to judge. We made a promise at the start of the book, and we believe we've delivered on it. We hope you can see that it would be very difficult for you to have any problem that this healing model will not address. If you have relationship problems, it's because somebody is not understanding the truth about the relationship, about your life, about circumstances or about themselves. But the issues that cause problems can be clarified by understanding the truth.

If you have a career or financial or achievement issue in your life, we can guarantee you that the thing that has been blocking your success is a misunderstanding of the truth. It causes us to not do the things that will result in achievement and success, and to do the things that will tend to sabotage our results. In other words, we're believing a lie that robs us of the power we need to succeed.

And, of course, if you have a health issue, according to the latest, greatest research from our greatest minds and medical schools, believing an untruth is always at the root of health problems. It triggers the stress response of the body, closes our cells, and we end up sick.

So if we have made good on our promise and you do see hope for your situation, your problem, or the fulfillment of your dream, then we challenge you to take the final step and turn one more page to learn about the mechanism that can create a new foundation for your life, health, and prosperity. In Part Two we're going to put it all together to show you exactly how to heal the stress that is causing your problems—both the unconscious stress from bad cellular memories, and the conscious stress from circumstances. You can start changing your life before the day is over.

PART TWO

Solutions:
How to Heal Virtually Any Health,
Relationship or Success Issue

CHAPTER NINE

What Is a Healing Code?

One of the most popular and published areas of self-help over the last forty years is the area of positive thinking, intention, coping, etc. While there is an element of truth in almost all of these approaches to a problem, there's also a critical element missing. I've already spoken about the library of self-help and psychology books in our living room; just about any popular self-help author you can name has been in Tracey's library. More than that, Tracey, being the perfectionist she is, tried each program, technique, or healing advice to the letter of the law. She was always still depressed.

You may be tempted to think this is an isolated situation. During my years of private practice counseling and therapy, however, I took an unofficial poll of my clients to get to the bottom of this issue. These are clients with problems ranging from major illness and disease to major mental illness to relationship struggles to all sorts of addictions. I would ask my clients two questions.

The first question was: "What should you be doing differently in relation to your problem?" Of the several hundred people I asked, only two did not know the correct answer. One was schizophrenic and the other was a rebellious teenager who I'm certain knew the right answer but was not going to tell me.

The second question was: "Why aren't you doing it?" Everyone's answer fell into one of two categories: "I don't know" or "I can't." All of these people—I repeat, *all of these people*—were trying as hard as they could to get over their problem or had tried at some time in the past, but were finally in the place of hopelessness. This finding is not an isolated one. Any counselor or therapist worth their salt will tell you about this phenomenon.

So why is it that these multimillion-dollar-selling books, techniques, and programs don't seem to work for the people who desperately need the help? Like most truth, the answer here is very simple. None of those things have the capacity to heal the source of the problem. What's my proof? If they did, the problems would be healed—not in just a few cases, but consistently and predictably for both physical and nonphysical issues.

How do I know that's even in the realm of possibility? First of all, because according to the theory and research, complete healing is what should happen (remember Secrets 1, 2, and 3), although historically, we've never had the mechanism to make it happen. More importantly, that's what our experience has been with The Healing Codes since their discovery in the spring of 2001.

In Chapter Two, you read several testimonials of people who have been healed. We are including more here to show you what's possible. These stories were unsolicited; they come from the lives that have been changed over the last eight or more years from 50 states and 90 countries. Any time you are ready to get on to the "what it is" and "how to" portion of this chapter, just to go to page 202 and get started.

Before you do, however, we would highly advise you to at least skim through the next few pages. Why? These are real people, just like you. Male, female, old, young, sick, healthy, hopeful, hopeless—all people who were searching as you are (or you wouldn't be reading this). We even have testimonials about pets and animals that have experienced miraculous healing. Our hope is that you find yourself in the next few pages and that it gives you hope to take action before another irretrievable day passes by.

By the way, you'll see in this book references to "The Healing Codes" or "The Healing Code" (plural or singular). "The Healing Codes" is a system that uses specific Codes for specific issues, covering any issue you can ever have in your life. The Healing Code is the one "Universal Healing Code" that we have discovered through years of testing works for just about anyone for just about any issue. They are both based on the same procedure and they both address the underlying heart issues. The testimonials are from people who have used either the system or The Healing Code in this book.

Healing Codes in Action: Testimonials from Users[17]

⚜

Unforgiveness

I was on vacation on the East Coast away from my husband. Starting The Healing Codes had really done me a lot of good. I felt different in general, even euphoric a lot of the time. I felt so much love for everyone. I felt different about everyone I was visiting. I saw them in a new light. For a long time I have had unforgiveness issues with my husband. I was at a "10" rating of my negative emotions toward him. As going home to him approached, this issue hung over me. I decided to refocus myself on unforgiveness with this issue in mind. When I arrived home, my husband and I sat down to talk and my negative emotions were gone! I was amazed since I had years of thinking that it couldn't change. This issue is now a 0! — Tena

17 For video testimonials, visit our site at www.thehealingcodebook.com.

Child's Fear of Parents' Death

My daughter Kelsey is ten years old. Ever since I can remember, she has always been insecure. Always needing much attention and basically very clingy. It has become unbearable over the last five or six months. My husband and I were at our wit's end and did not know what to do. Kelsey has been obsessed with death for a long time. She has had nightmares, sleepless nights, days of crying, unable to go to school and an overall terrible experience because she thought either my husband or I was going to die.

My sister-in-law encouraged us to try The Healing Codes on her. I wasn't sure how to approach it with my daughter and tried to keep it very simple. She seemed very open, so I asked her to picture one of the pictures that have been bothering her. She did, started crying and rated it a 10. She picked her truth statements and I started the Healing Codes for peace on her. She started deep breathing and relaxing immediately. I didn't think she would sit still because she is usually very fidgety. She just sat there relaxed. When we were finished she was already very different. I was so excited. She said her picture [memory] was almost a 0 and she seemed very happy. She kept asking me to do them with her. The next time she picked a different picture and also rated it a 10. Again after that she said the picture didn't bother her anymore. She doesn't have any more pictures and feels great. She is a different little girl. Praise God for the Healing Codes. I have witnessed a miracle in my daughter. — Sue

∽✥∾

Scoliosis and Chronic Pain

I've had scoliosis since I was seven, and I wore a body cast for about five years. By the time I hit my twenties, I was in chronic pain. Over the years, I've done chiropractic work, yoga, body work, supplements, and the list goes on. It was always very momentary relief. I guess I never handled and processed stress very well, so everything was a trigger from my external world and felt overwhelming. From the first time I did a Code, I felt dramatic results. First I felt this deep relaxation and a sense of peace. All my body pain was gone, and I felt much lighter and more calm, focused and fluid in my body movements. It's been thirty years that I've had this body pain, and now I'm free of it.

I've been doing The Healing Codes for about two and a half months now. My lungs are clearing out, there is a lot of detoxing, and my spine is straightening. Some of the bones that had fused from the stress of the scoliosis are now starting to open up. Huge changes! I'd been down to working three days a week because I couldn't handle more, and it would take me almost three days to recover. Now I come home from work after three days and I feel great. I'm ready to enjoy life, and I seem to be handling the stress much differently. Thank you for the wonderful self-healing technique, Dr. Loyd, and thank you for sharing it with everyone. — Katherine

∽◌∾

Regained Functioning Years after Surgery

My husband and I have been doing The Healing Codes together for about three months now. We're finding that we're not only feeling so much better generally, we're happier, more outgoing, and more confident than we were. Even after fifty years of marriage there's still a lot for us to learn and to do together. My husband had a bout with cancer about three and a half to four years ago. He had to have major surgery on the left side of his face and suffered through the radiation. He lost the sense of feeling and the ability to produce saliva, and lost a great deal of ability to taste. Those things are beginning to come back now. He has feeling on the left side of his head, and he is able to taste things that he hasn't been able to taste for years. The dry mouth is going away. I swear he's growing more hair on the top of his bald head! The doctors had said that he'd improved as much as he was going to. But with The Codes, he has improved even more, and we're really excited about it. We feel very blessed.

— Marilyn

Emotional and Behavioral Healing (Addiction)

I was aware The Healing Codes were used in the beginning for emotional issues, and you later began to discover them working on physical issues as well. I purchased the Codes to use for a physical issue. The irony has been to see that the more diligent I am to do the Codes for my physical issue the more emotional healing I experience. I have received excellent counseling and been a part of 12-Step groups. Even though I know I have experienced much healing from those modalities, The Healing Codes have taken healthy behavior for me from a conscious thought process to an automatic behavior. It is a whole new level of freedom and for that I am very grateful. — Jamie

Insomnia

Let me say how happy I am with the Codes. I almost instantly changed my sleep pattern. I have had problems with insomnia on and off almost my whole life and I now sleep better and harder than I ever have before. I keep doing the Codes and trust that this will heal the other problems I have as well. — Helle

Extreme Pain (Trigeminal Neuralgia)

For over eight years I have experienced the pain caused by a condition called trigeminal neuralgia. This is extreme facial pain triggered by eating, talking, brushing teeth, touching ... or just a slight breeze on the cheek. Sometimes I would just be lying perfectly still and experience repeated sharp lacerating facial pain. Even when I was not experiencing pain, I constantly lived in expectation/fear of the next series of lightning-like bolts of pain.

After just two weeks of using the Healing Codes, I sensed that there was a lessening of pain, both intensity and frequency. In another week, I experienced a day and a half pain free ... and after that a steady, gradual reduction in the intensity and frequency of pain. It is two months since I began, and I am thrilled to tell the world that I have been totally pain free for the past week. This is so amazing!! I will continue to use the Codes daily for the rest of my life!! Thank you all! — Sarah

∽✃

Back Injury and Migraines

I hurt my back very badly by lifting a toolbox that I really knew was too heavy. After a couple of days the pain in my back had really become unbearable and had traveled down my leg. I went to two different chiropractors, but this time they couldn't help me at all. I then called my doctor, and she gave me a prescription for pain and a muscle relaxer, and then had me do physical therapy for six weeks. Nothing helped. A dear friend told me about The Healing Codes and I ordered them. I was ready to try anything. In a few short days I was on the mend, and after a week I no longer had the pain. I couldn't believe it. I encouraged my husband to try them and see how they would work for him. He has had some success with his migraines. Now he is using them for hypoglycemia. — Joyce

∽✃

Diabetes

For the last ten years I have been an insulin dependent diabetic, and have had to inject insulin four times a day. What was beginning to worry me were the diabetic complications that were starting to show. The first was very cold hands and feet, second was small problems with the eyes, aching legs, getting up three or four times a night to go for a wee, feeling tired all the time, loosing my temper and getting stressed very easily.

So OK, you're saying, what's improved? Well I've been doing this program at home for three weeks now. So far the leg ache has gone, and the legs feel so much lighter when walking uphill. I notice a world of difference, no longer getting up in the middle of the night, no longer feeling tired. I'm starting to get more feeling in my feet and they are no longer cold. The one thing everybody else in my family noticed very quickly was that I was no longer losing my temper, and have been very calm for me, not getting stressed out over the slightest thing. Have I healed myself from diabetes? At this time I would say no, not yet. But what I will say is that I have had to reduce the insulin that I'm injecting, because my sugar levels are dropping. I have only been doing the Codes for four weeks now, and I feel better than I've felt in ten to fifteen years. — Steve

Pet Healed

I have been doing The Healing Codes for several months now with good results but nothing like what I experienced last night. I have many exotic animals in my home and last night I got home from work late and had to take care of these guys much faster than usual. One of my small lizards was out and about and I did not notice her until I accidentally stepped on her head.

She was bleeding from the mouth and her eye and I felt that her skull was crushed. I felt so bad. She was limp with blood coming out of her mouth. I thought she was dead at this point. I laid her on some paper towels and thought about the Codes, and did one for her for 45 minutes. I kept checking on her. Her breathing was very shallow and she was not conscious. In two hours she was back up to her normal self but kept her eye closed. By the next day she had both eyes open and was acting as usual. Thank you all so much for this incredible process.—Bill

Cancer

When my best friend and sweetheart learned she had metastatic melanoma I helped her begin to use The Healing Codes along with her very strict diet to bring her immune system into balance. Her recent CAT-scans showed her to be completely cancer free. We are anxiously awaiting the next blood test that will show her having a balanced immune system. — William

❦

Healing for Family Members (Hemorrhoids)

Through the years, I have dealt with healing issues in a number of ways with some limited success—EFT, Sedona Method, HoloSynch, Theta Healing, Chi Gong, nutritionals—I have even tried hypnosis.

So you can see, I have always believed and searched for a way to find inner peace, and a way to heal myself. I knew someday—I would find the ONE KEY to healing myself and my loved ones. Well, I found my KEY. It is this: **The Healing Codes!**

I have released lifelong erroneous beliefs that do not serve me, some which have impacted me in areas of my career, my health and emotional stability—and **it has been easy!** I have lost weight without trying to. I have even been able to help those whom I love to be relieved of their health issues!

One of these issues has been my husband's hemorrhoids. He has lived with them for over twenty years, and they have really bothered him for the past few years. I finally got him to agree to see a doctor about this, but the soonest the specialist could see him was three months out. So, I started doing Codes for him!

The day of his appointment, he told me he didn't think he needed to go, as he thought the hemorrhoids had cleared up. I thought he was just trying to get out of going to the doctor, so I insisted he keep the appointment—in fact, I went with him! Get this! The hemorrhoid specialist could not find any evidence of hemorrhoids! He did not even know why my husband was there. He asked the nurse to check too. Nothing. My husband was shocked and asked, "Are you sure?" No treatment was necessary, and he was given a clean bill of health!

My husband now asks me every day to do Codes for this or that—and I always do!

So, I can say my search is over, I have found the Key to healing on *all levels, body, mind, spirit. If anyone doubts, I say just try this with an open heart, and you too will be a believer! — Laurie*

∽⚬∾

Miracles or Just a New Paradigm?

Do all these healings sound like miracles? If so, then consider this quote by St. Augustine: "Miracles happen, not in opposition to Nature, but in opposition to what we know of Nature." God built the possibility of "miraculous" healing into us at creation as part of his original intention for the world, and it is still available to us today. The Healing Codes have just been discovered recently, by God's grace, but the mechanism for healing has always been in us. Perhaps the reason it's only been discovered recently is that, until the past few years, we have not had the science nor the metaphors for understanding how it works. What was formerly hidden, because we just did not have the capacity to understand, has now been brought to light because of other recent advances.

So now, let's get down to it: How and why does a Healing Code work?

THE PHYSICAL MECHANISM THAT DEACTIVATES STRESS

As we've described throughout this book, stress is the source of all our ills. A Healing Code works by getting rid of stress at the source. Research from the Institute of HeartMath in California indicates that if the stress can be removed, even the genes will often heal. They identified an internal healing resource so powerful it literally has a healing effect on damaged DNA.

The discovery of The Healing Codes revealed the physical function that automatically activates that healing resource identified by the Institute of HeartMath. Using this healing resource, *a Healing Code heals by changing the underlying destructive energy pattern, or frequency, of a destructive image to a healthy one.*

Healing energy, directed at different combinations of the four healing centers on the body, is used to heal different unhealthy beliefs and images. These healing combinations could be compared to the four nucleotides that make up our DNA. Every difference in every person in the world is determined by a unique combination of just four nucleotides.

This fits beautifully with recent research findings that our memories and images may literally be stored in the energy information field of every cell of the body, similarly to DNA. (This would also explain why organ transplant patients may experience memories of the donor.) When you do a Healing Code with the appropriate combination of the four healing centers, we believe that you are literally showering every cell in the body with healthy healing energy.

So what exactly is a Healing Code, and how can it activate such a profound process?

THE FOUR HEALING CENTERS

The discovery of The Healing Codes is really the discovery of four healing centers on the body. The four healing centers of the body correspond to the master control centers for every cell in the body. These healing centers appear to work like a hidden fuse box that, when the correct switches are flipped on, will allow healing of almost anything. They do this by removing the stress in the body that had switched them off, thus allowing the neuro-immune system to resume its job of healing whatever is wrong in the body.

If you follow the path of the healthy energy as it travels through the four healing centers into the body, the physical systems you would discover would include:

Bridge: The pituitary gland (often referred to as the master gland because it controls the major endocrine processes of the body) and the pineal gland.

Temples: The higher functioning left and right brain, and the hypothalamus.

Jaw: The reactive emotional brain, including the amygdala and hippocampus, plus the spinal cord and the central nervous system.

Adam's Apple: The spinal cord and central nervous system, plus the thyroid.

In other words, *you would discover the control centers for every system, every organ, and every cell of the body.* Healing energy from these centers flows to them all.

HOW A HEALING CODE ACTIVATES
THE HEALING CENTERS

You activate the healing centers with your fingers. A Healing Code is one set of easy hand positions. It's very simple. We can teach a child of six or seven how to do it easily. You perform a Healing Code by aiming all five fingers of both hands at one or more of the healing centers from two to three inches away from the body. The hands and fingers direct flows of energy at the healing centers.

The healing centers activate an energetic healing system that functions in a manner parallel to the immune system. Instead of killing viruses and bacteria, it targets memories related to the issue a person is thinking about. Using positive, healing energy frequencies, it cancels out and replaces the negative, destructive frequencies.

When cells are showered with healthy energy by doing a Healing Code, the unhealthy energy is literally cancelled by the positive energy, similarly to the way noise cancellation headphones cancel harmful sound frequencies. After the destructive frequencies are cancelled, the image will resonate with healthy energy that will contribute to the good health of the cells, organs, and body system that it resides in. Healing energy has transformed destructive energy that was stored as cellular memories in the body/mind, ultimately affecting the physiology of the cells in the body.

WHY IS IT A "CODE"?

The reason we call it "The Healing Codes" is that every procedure involves a coded sequence. When the two of us lectured in Maui, we were fortunate to have a key to the door, in the form of a code. The front door had a keypad with a four-digit code, so when we came up to the door we punched in that code ("beep beep beep beep") and we heard a click as the door unlocked. Perhaps you have a garage door opener that works in a similar way.

That's kind of how The Healing Codes work. The exercise turns on some combination of those four healing centers in a priority sequence. The priority sequence is critical to remove the stress in the body related to a particular problem and to heal the cellular memories related to that problem. The average Healing Code takes about 6 minutes to do, activating those healing centers with your fingers. You can do it comfortably while lying down in a recliner. We've had reports of people doing it while they're talking on the phone, watching TV, reading a book, and other activities.

The Healing Code we will give you in the next chapter activates all of the four healing centers in the optimal sequence, and we believe that is why it seems to work on almost every issue for almost every person.

IS THERE EVIDENCE THAT THE HEALING CODES REALLY WORK?

As described earlier, the validity of The Healing Codes is established by:

1. Thousands of clients' reports of self-healing from all manner of problems, including many regarded as incurable.

2. Mainstream diagnostic tests (Heart Rate Variability) showing stress is consistently removed from the body following the use of a Healing Code.

This is a relatively new method, and the validation of our results is still a work in progress, as is our understanding of how a Healing Code works.

This is not at all unusual, even for things that have been used for decades by millions of people. For instance, we may not have a clue as to how particular medicines work, but we believe they do, and so we take them. You may be surprised to know that researchers are uncertain of the way many common medicines work, despite years—even decades or more—of their use. The following are just a few examples out of the *Physicians Desk Reference* (PDR), a primary reference used by physicians to guide them in prescribing pharmaceutical drugs:

Accutane: "The exact mechanism of Accutane is unknown."

Zoloft: "The mechanism of sertraline [Zoloft] is *presumed* to be linked to its inhibition of CNS neuronal uptake of serotonin." [Emphasis added.]

Xanax: "Exact mechanism of action is unknown."

Risperdal: "The mechanism of Risperdal, like all other anti-psychotics, is unknown."

Depakote: "The mechanism by which valproate [Depakote] exerts its therapeutic effects has not been established."

The above is a representative sample from several major categories of drugs. The PDR is filled with many other drugs whose method of action is also unknown or uncertain.

WHAT SEEMS LIKE A MIRACLE IS SIMPLY A NEW DISCOVERY

Let us repeat the words of St. Augustine: "Miracles happen, not in opposition to Nature, but in opposition to what we know of Nature."

Although we have known for a long time that destructive energy patterns cause stress and health problems, little is being done by modern medicine to resolve these patterns. The reason you haven't heard more about these truths is that no one has found a reliable, consistent, predictable, validated way to change destructive energy patterns to healthy ones in the body. Moreover, even attempting to do so does not fit the paradigm of traditional modern medicine, which is focused on biochemical treatment, not prevention or healing using bio-energy.

According to physics, the exact equal and opposite frequency is required to cancel out another frequency. For a Healing Code to work, something has to find the related unconscious memories, and something has to determine their frequencies, and something has to create the equal and opposite frequencies. And it does!

It not only works, it seems to work almost 100 percent of the time. At a conference in Mexico, 142 out of 142 who did a Healing Code on a memory related to the biggest issue of their lives had the negative power of that memory heal down to a zero or 1 on a 10 point scale. With results like this, we have to be tapping into a system that is designed to heal. If something happened over 99 percent of the time in nature, we wouldn't even need to do a study. We know an object will fall every time we drop it, and we believed this long before we understood the invisible force of gravity.

Not only does it work, but the effects last. As mentioned, the Heart Rate Variability studies showed that people remained in balance long after they had done the Healing Code. When tested against systems that use the chakra/meridian(acupuncture points) energy system, HRV tests showed people using both methods got their autonomic nervous systems in balance immediately (about 7 out of 10 with meridians, about 8 out of 10 with Healing Codes). However, twenty-four hours later, only 2 out of 10 of the meridian protocol people stayed in balance, while more than 7 out of 10 of The Healing Codes users remained in balance. These results had never been seen before, we were told.

Based on our experience and research, we believe that healing these destructive energy patterns is precisely what a Healing Code does. And the news is even better than that! *A*

Healing Code works without our having to be consciously aware of the destructive images, beliefs, thoughts and feelings that are being healed.

A Healing Code—that works exclusively on the destructive memory pictures in the heart—is able to heal the stress and the wrong beliefs that underlie the physical and non-physical problems in our lives.

We may not be able to explain it fully yet, but we do believe we know the nature of the seemingly miraculous healing energy that is accessed by a Healing Code.

WHAT IS THIS AMAZING HEALING ENERGY?

Just as all colors of light are contained in pure white light, similarly we believe that all virtues are contained in pure love (courage, truth, loyalty, joy, peace, patience, etc.).

In fact, *we believe that the energy frequency of pure love will heal anything—and that it may be the only power that will.* The vibrational frequency of love is the ultimate healing resource.

WHAT IS OUR SCIENTIFIC BASIS FOR THIS THEORY?

In the last few years several individuals have been able to isolate and quantify the frequencies of love and other virtues. The frequency of love resides in us in every loving memory of our heart. Let me prove it to you.

Think about the most joyful, loving memory of your life. Take a moment to fully relive this memory with your eyes closed, calling it back into life again. What do you feel? Don't you feel good? Don't you re-experience, at least to some degree, the loving event—even if it occurred decades ago? Why does that happen?

The instant you access and activate a loving memory, the frequency of love is transmitted throughout your body, and it has a corresponding physiological healing effect. As mentioned earlier, the Institute of HeartMath has published studies indicating that activating these types of positive memories can actually have a healing effect on damaged DNA.[18]

In the same way that our loving memories transmit healing frequencies all over our bodies, painful, destructive and distorted memories transmit frequencies that cause illness and disease. According to Dr. Lipton's research, these destructive memories broadcast a signal in the body that causes us to interpret current circumstances as threatening even when they aren't. This is what keeps our body under stress. I encourage you to do an experiment with this as well. Recall a memory that is still painful for you and notice how you feel. If you think of this memory long enough, you will not only feel bad, you will literally shift your cells into the "self-protection mode" and your nervous system into "fight-or-flight."

Unfortunately, your unconscious mind can be focused on these destructive images without your ever knowing it. When this happens, it has the same damaging effect to the physiology of your body as conscious negative thoughts and images. Many people walk around every day with this "process of creating illness and disease" occurring, and they never know it until they become very ill. This is why the source of our problems is unconscious at least 90 percent of the time, making it impossible to consciously address the cause of our physical, emotional and spiritual issues.

---

18 See www.heartmath.com.

The good news is that *the key to healing issues at their root is found inside the human heart*, not in anything outside of us. All that is needed is a way to take the power of the love resources of the heart and use them to heal the destructive images that lead to illness.

WHY CAN'T YOU HEAL ON YOUR OWN?

If the love resources are already inside us broadcasting their healing signals, why don't these images heal on their own?

This gets us back to Secret #5. The problem is that there are certain memories or images that seem to be guarded from receiving healing when healing frequencies are broadcast all over the body. This may be a hidden or repressed memory, as described in psychology, but we might also be completely aware of the memory. It is as if the mind has literally built a fort or stronghold around certain memories. It does this to protect us from the pain of something similar happening to us again. It believes that if we aren't vigilantly on guard, we might be hurt again. Preventing pain is fine, but by protecting the destructive images in this way, the mind can also prevent the resources of the body from reaching and healing the destructive images. What is needed is a way to infuse healing frequencies into the images that are causing the problem but are not receiving the healing energy.

This is precisely what a Healing Code does. By accessing the love and healthy resources from all over the body, the Healing Code then transmits those frequencies through the fingers into the four healing centers to change the energy patterns from destructive images to healthy ones, even the ones being guarded.

People tell us over and over again that as they do The Healing Code, hurtful memories seem to just melt away and, as they do, physical symptoms also disappear. I believe this is exactly what those physicists were predicting when they made comments such as that of Dr. William Tiller, who said, "Future medicine will be based on controlling energy frequencies in the body."

With that, we welcome you to try The Healing Code. May it change your life as it has changed ours and so many others' lives!

∽◦∾

Sports and Peak Performance

As a professional athlete, I have been on TV, magazine covers, newspaper headlines, et cetera. I left home at an early age to train to be a world-class professional athlete—and I became just that. I have tried all the peak performance psychology and training available, the highest-priced doctors in New York and Los Angeles.

Everything else tries to teach you to "cope" with what is limiting you, or just ignore it with the use of some mental trick—tricks that don't work most of the time and take a great deal of effort. The Healing Code does what nothing else does: It fixes the source of what is holding you back or limiting you, and it empowers you to excel to your maximum capabilities! Best of all, the Code does this quickly and simply, in a way that is almost effortless. IT LITERALLY REPROGRAMS YOU FOR SUCCESS!—Michael, Los Angeles

Disclaimer & Informed Consent

The Healing Code and Instant Impact are for informational and educational purposes only. Neither is intended to diagnose, prescribe, treat, or cure any disease or mental condition. The FDA has not evaluated this information and we make no curative claims.

Testimonials represent a cross section of the range of results that appear to be typical with these products. Results may vary depending upon use and commitment. Individuals who have provided their testimonial are not compensated in any way.

All Healing Codes techniques—including The Universal Healing Code and the Instant Impact exercise included in this book—are self-help techniques used for relaxation, stress reduction, and balancing bio-energetic systems, and are not intended as a substitute for medical care. No action or inaction should be taken based solely on the contents herein; instead, readers or viewers should consult appropriate health professionals on any matter relating to their health. The Healing Code addresses what Solomon called "issues of the heart" more than 3000 years ago. There is no Code for any physical or mental disease or illness; every Healing Code focuses only on the spiritual issues of the heart. When these spiritual issues heal, physiological stress reduces, and the immune system functioning increases. The immune system is capable of healing just about anything if it is not suppressed by stress. Our focus 100 percent of the time with The Healing Code is for the issues of the heart—only.

The Healing Code is also NOT counseling or therapy of any kind. It is the application of a healing tool discovered in 2001 and first offered to the public in 2004. Any Healing Code targets only the destructive pictures of the heart (memories) and is intended to be used only as directed. Sporadic or non-committal use of this Code may slow the picture-healing process. No one is advised to discontinue or avoid medical or psychological consultations.

The Healing Code theory and practice are based on experience. After the discovery of *The Healing Codes®* system in 2001, we tested it for one and a half years, and then spent one and a half years packaging it so that anyone can easily do it for themselves at home. It is unique and one of a kind. We have never had one person who reported to us that they had seen this before.

According to Paul Harris, PhD, "this is the only health field where there has never in history been a validated case of harm." Although this literature and our results reflect our experiences, your results cannot be guaranteed. What you can reasonably expect by doing The Healing Code is that the issues of your heart will heal or improve, and by doing Instant Impact, that your feelings of stress will decrease.

Accordingly, this book and the methods it describes should not be substituted for the advice and treatment of a physician or other licensed health-care professional. This information and the opinions provided here are believed to be accurate and sound, based on the best knowledge, experience, and research of the authors. Readers who fail to consult with appropriate health authorities assume the risk of any injuries.

Using the techniques herein is acknowledging that you have read, understand, and agree to this disclaimer and, therefore, that informed consent has been established.

CHAPTER TEN

Your 6-Minute "Universal Healing Code"

Throughout this book, we have been referring to The Healing Codes® because that is what I discovered in 2001, and that is what our data is based on.

In working with thousands of clients, doing live presentations, and testing, we have come to the conclusion that there is indeed one Healing Code that seems to work for almost everyone, on almost any issue. Probably because it activates all of the four healing centers, this one Healing Code acts as sort of the "master Code" to unlock healing for stress of any kind.

It will only take you a few minutes to learn this Healing Code, but the results will last you a lifetime!

Remember that you can do this for other people, even pets, as well. Just follow the instructions!

A WORD ABOUT PRAYER

The Healing Code incorporates prayer. Prayer is one of the most studied practices in medicine. Over and over it has been proven that prayer helps people heal—even if they don't pray themselves but are prayed for by others. Prayer is always my first course of action, even before I do any Healing Code. The Healing Code is just a tool, an amazing new "screwdriver" that does things no other screwdriver has ever done before. Still, it's just a screwdriver. What's most important is your relationship with God, however you work that out. So we urge you to make prayer your primary focus, using The Healing Code as part of the process. (One client says The Healing Code "puts prayer on steroids.")

HOW TO DO THE UNIVERSAL HEALING CODE

Use the four exercise positions shown below in the order they are listed, and "shine" your relaxed fingers at the healing centers (as though your fingertips are little flashlights clustered together) two to three inches off the body. It doesn't matter if your fingers are straight or curved (whatever is most comfortable for you), only that the fingertips are aimed at the area surrounding the healing center.

Having your fingertips two to three inches away from the body is several times more effective than touching the healing centers with the fingers. It creates an energy field over the entrance of the healing center that allows the body to automatically produce the precise positive/negative energy pattern needed for healing. The reason for the increased effectiveness crystallized for me while we were doing a seminar in Oklahoma City. A gentleman shared that having the fingers away from the body makes perfect sense: it works just like a spark plug. I'm no mechanic, but he said that the spark plug doesn't touch the metal. There is a gap there and the energy arcs from the spark plug to the metal. He said that in fact, if there's not enough of a gap, it won't work right. There won't be enough power. The same is true of The Healing Code. Having the fingers away from the body creates the exact polarity needed at any given second to give significantly greater power.

The Four Healing Centers

Bridge: In between the bridge of the nose and the middle of the eyebrow, if the eyebrows were grown together

Adam's Apple: Directly over the Adam's apple

Jaws: On the bottom back corner of the jawbone, on both sides of the head

Temples: One half inch above the temple, and one half inch toward the back of the head, on both sides of the head

Each of the four healing centers has a normal hand position and a resting hand position except the Adam's apple; the normal position for that is a resting position. The resting positions are provided so you can rest your hands on your body and do the procedures more comfortably. As mentioned, for the normal positions, your fingertips are two to three inches off the body from the healing center. For the resting positions, your fingertips aim across the top of the healing center from two to three inches below or beside the center.

Add a few minutes to the Code when using the resting positions. If your arms become too fatigued to perform a Code for the specified amount of time, try the resting positions, or prop your arms up with a pillow, or rest your elbows on a table or desk. **If your hands drift off the center, healing will still occur. Your intention to heal is far more important than being perfect at holding the hand positions.**

It is helpful to rate how much discomfort you feel when thinking about your issue or problem on a scale from 0 to 10 (10 being the most discomfort) before doing The Healing Code. This is the best way to measure your progress as you see the discomfort level decrease until it reaches a 0 or 1.

Do the Code in a quiet, private, place where you can relax without distractions or interruptions.

Here's the sequence:

1. Rate the issue in terms of how much it bothers you, 0-10, 10 being most painful.

2. Identify the feelings and/or unhealthy beliefs related to your issue.

3. Memory Finder: Think back if there was another time in your life when you felt the same way, even if the circumstances were very different. We're looking for the same kind of feeling. Don't do a lot of digging—just take a moment to ask yourself if there was another time in your life when you felt the same way you're feeling now. We're going for similarities in the feeling, not the circumstances. If you're feeling anxious about an upcoming medical test, you want to ask if you have ever felt that same kind of anxiety when you were younger, not whether you ever faced a medical test before. Go for the earliest memory that surfaces, and focus on healing that first.

4. Rate that earlier memory, 0-10. There may be others. Look for the strongest or earliest, and work on that first. What bothers us now tends to be troublesome precisely because it's attached to or triggered by an unhealed memory. Often when you heal the earlier or strongest memory, all other memories "attached" to that core memory heal at the same time.

5. Say the prayer for healing, inserting all the issues you uncovered ("my memory as a four-year-old, my fear issue, my headaches," or whatever).

"I pray that all known and unknown negative images, unhealthy beliefs, destructive cellular memories, and all physical issues related to _____ [your problem or issues] would be found, opened and healed by filling me with the light, life and love of God. I also pray that the effectiveness of this healing be increased by 100 times or more." (This tells the body to make the healing a priority.)

6. Do The Healing Code holding each position for around 30 seconds, repeating a Truth Focus Statement[19] that counters any unhealthy belief, or one that addresses your issue. When you do a Healing Code, you don't focus on the negative, but the positive. Make sure you rotate through all four positions before quitting (usually several sequences). **Do the Code sequence for at least 6 minutes.** Make sure you go through all four positions before you stop. You can always take a little longer, especially if you rated your issue above a 5 or 6. We suggest 6 minutes as the minimum.

(First Position) Bridge: In between the bridge of the nose and the middle of the eyebrow, if the eyebrows were grown together.

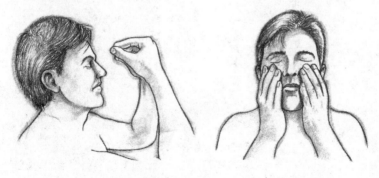

Main Bridge position   Resting

19 One of your bonuses when you register the book is access to sample Truth Focus Statements. www.thehealingcodebook.com

(Second Position) Adam's Apple: Directly over the Adam's apple.

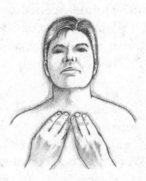

(Third Position) Jaws: On the bottom back corner of the jawbone, on both sides of the head.

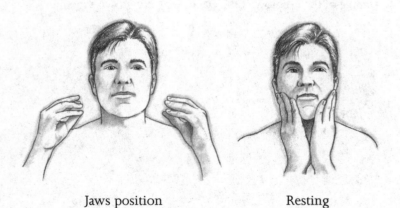

Jaws position   Resting

(Fourth Position) Temples: One half inch above the temple, and one half inch toward the back of the head, on both sides of the head.

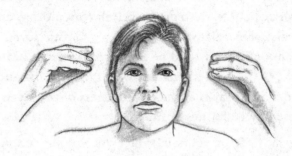

Temples

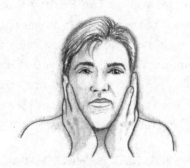

Resting

7. After doing the Code, rate your issue again. When that earliest/strongest memory is down to 0 or 1, you can go on to the next memory or issue that bothers you the most.

DOING THE CODE FOR SOMEONE ELSE

You can do The Healing Code on behalf of someone else. Simply say the prayer, like this:

"I pray that all known and unknown negative images, unhealthy beliefs, destructive cellular memories, and all physical issues related to _____ [your loved one's problem or issue] would be found, opened and healed by filling _____ [person's name] with the light, life and love of God. I also pray that the effectiveness of this healing be increased by 100 times or more."

Do the Code on yourself. When you're done, simply pray, "I release the full effects of this healing to [name of person], in love."

We recommend you do The Healing Code three times a day. You can do it more as needed, to get faster results. You may still get results with doing it just once a day, and we strongly recommend you make sure you do it at least once a day. You can also do it longer than 6 minutes. *Consistency is key.* Doing it for 6 minutes three times or more times a day is ideal, and will give you the best results.

QUESTIONS YOU MAY HAVE ABOUT DOING THE HEALING CODE

What should I expect to happen when I do my Healing Code?

There are two areas in which you will most likely see a change or shift when you do The Healing Code:

1. The picture or memory you are focusing on.
2. The physical or non-physical problem resulting from the memories.

Changes to your memory picture: Keep in mind that The Healing Code heals only the pictures in the heart. It does not remove pictures from the memory. This means that the emotional intensity attached to the memory picture is removed, not the picture itself. Many people report that as they use the Code, the picture that they are focusing on begins to fade, and often becomes hard to visualize and hold in focus. As the memory is healed, some individuals describe it as if the energy of power has been drained out of the picture, and that it doesn't control them anymore. There is often an accompanying feeling of peace and closure. You will know that your picture is healed when you experience some or perhaps all of the signs mentioned here.

Changes to the issue bothering you the most: As your picture heals, you will usually begin to see a change in other issues that are bothering you. However, it is important to understand that while some issues have only one picture attached to them, some may have many more than that. If, after completing the Code on a particular picture, your most bothersome issue is unchanged, don't be discouraged. If you continue the process of working on your images, healing will occur within the capability of your immune system to heal the problem.

In our live seminars when we do The Healing Code with people, they consistently report feeling a difference in one 6-minute session. Obviously issues such as cancer may take many 6-minute sessions. So when we say "6 minutes to heal any issue" we mean it in the same way you would say, "Take Vitamin C to fight colds and boost your immune system." Everybody knows that doesn't mean "take one Vitamin C one time and you'll never get a cold." It means if you take Vitamin

C consistently, you are likely to get colds and other illnesses less frequently. The Healing Code works just like that—it works when you do it consistently.

What if I feel like I am not making much progress?

If you feel that you are working and not making progress, focus on the picture of when the problem started and when the physical and non-physical symptoms began. For example, if migraines have you physically in pain and emotionally depressed, focus on when the pain and depression started.

If, after doing the Code five separate times, you still have not felt any reduction in the 0 to 10 intensity rating, look again for another picture. This may be a picture between your earliest one and the current picture, or it may be your current picture. Work on the picture of greatest intensity instead of the earliest time.

You might also try going to the time in your life shortly before your problem started (up to two years before). You will sometimes find a shock, trauma, or intense emotional event in this time period. Focus on this event until its emotions and beliefs are healed.

If you still do not experience a change in your condition, it may be because another issue is tied to the root of your current problem. Continue working on the issues and category bothering you most until the problem breaks. (In the next chapter, we will tell you about a tool we are making available that can help you pinpoint your issues. This can help especially if you don't feel you're making progress. Often what we think is the real issue isn't truly at the heart of the problem.)

What if I feel worse after completing my Code?

Uncomfortable healing responses occur with perhaps 1 in 10 people. It's not unique to using The Healing Codes. It is a well-known phenomenon in medicine called the Herxheimer reaction. We call this a healing response because it is evidence that you are indeed healing. Physical toxins and negative emotions may be working their way out of your system.

When you heal the destructive cellular memories and unhealthy beliefs that caused your issues, the resulting stress in your body will diminish. As this occurs, your neuro-immune system will start to heal the physiology of your body. During this process, toxins, viruses, and bacteria will often start to leave your body. When this happens, sometimes you will feel worse until the detoxification is complete. If you have used a detoxification regimen, you may recognize the symptoms. Drinking plenty of water will speed up the ability of your body to rid itself of toxins.

It's important to remember that *this is not a problem you are feeling—you are feeling your problems being healed!* It is one of the most wonderful things that can happen to you physiologically. However, it can also be uncomfortable. The most common healing responses that our clients report are headaches, fatigue, and a worsening of the feelings of the problems they are trying to heal. There is no rule, but generally the more junk that you have in your body or your heart, the more junk has to come out. Emotional issues are commonly a part of healing responses.

Healing responses are natural. We tend to think of the flu as fever, chills, sore throat, etc. This is not the flu at all; these are the healing responses of the body and immune system as it attempts to eliminate the virus that threatens it. The flu is the virus itself. You need not be alarmed then if you experience a healing response as the body gears into action to heal destructive images and the resulting stress on your physiology.

A healing response is evidence that you are progressing! It will stop when cleansing is complete.

Do I continue to do the Healing Code if I have a healing response?

Yes. If you have a healing response, continue with doing the Code, but shift your focus to easing the discomfort of the healing response.

Of course, if you have a symptom that you believe may be an illness or injury, seek the appropriate medical assistance.

According to Paul Harris, PhD, energy medicine is the only area of health where there has never been a validated case of harm. This is further evidence that the healing responses some people experience are part of a wonderful healing event, not a symptom of their problems.

As healing occurs, it is also not unusual to experience a back-and-forth response with your emotions. There may be days when you feel like "it's a miracle" or "I haven't felt this good in years," only to be followed by a day that reminds you of how you felt before the healing started. This too is normal. Try not to become impatient with the process. It takes as long as it takes. Remember, you are most likely healing decades of junk.

Example: We had two middle-aged male clients who had both suffered with migraine headaches for about fifteen years. One man's headaches healed within a week and never returned, while the other man took a year to heal. Why the huge time difference for the same problem? *Because they did not have the same problem!* They merely had the same symptoms. The Healing Code heals the spiritual source of a problem, which is always destructive cellular memories/images and unhealthy beliefs, not the physical symptoms, illness or disease. Although these two men had the same symptoms, they had radically different images as sources of their problems.

Should I quit taking medications? Will they interfere with The Healing Code?

Absolutely not! This is not meant to take the place of what you are now doing. Use this in addition to other healing aids. The Healing Code has been proven to work no matter what else you are doing for your problem. Never discontinue medications without consulting a healthcare professional.

Should I forgo medical treatment to do The Healing Code?

Absolutely not! The Healing Code is complementary and works well with traditional care. We believe you should do healing work from as many different healthy angles as possible. Never forego medical treatment or discontinue it without consulting a healthcare professional.

How will I know if this is working?

You may notice a deeper level of peace and relaxation. You may notice that the things you usually struggle with aren't difficult anymore. Or you may not recognize anything changing. The best way to observe your changes is to keep a record of the intensity ratings in the Memory Picture Finder. As those numbers decrease, you will know the Code is definitely working. You can download a free Tracking Chart when you register your book (www.thehealingcodebook.com).

How long will it take to get results?

Times required for healing vary dramatically from person to person. This is because seemingly identical problems (fear, headaches, etc.) can be caused by a variety of destructive memory pictures in different people, as mentioned in the above example concerning headaches.

What if I get interrupted during my session?

If you are interrupted when doing the Code, you may continue where you left off if you are interrupted once. If you are interrupted twice, start the Code again.

How closely should I watch the clock while doing my Code?

Try to do each position for an equal amount of time within the time allotted for the Code (at least 6 minutes). However, don't be distracted by a clock. The most important thing is your intention to heal and how it is affecting your pictures. If you use Truth Focus Statements[20] as suggested, you can time how many times amount to 30 seconds or so, and then just use that for your 30-second "timer."

How far apart should I do my sessions?

It is best to space your Healing Code sessions throughout the day. However, it is better to do them all at the same time, back to back, than to miss doing one.

How important is it to do each position exactly as it is pictured or described?

Try to do each position in the way it is described and pictured. However, if you are close it will work. The intention to heal is an important factor in success.

---

20 When you register your book at www.thehealingcodebook.com, you will have access to sample Truth Focus Statements.

Will the Code work on problems I am not focused on?

You may experience benefits outside of the issue you are working on at the time because different problems may be affected by the same picture.

Sometimes I feel like I have a battle going on inside myself. Why is that?

We call this *conscious conflict*. If something in your life violates your own belief system, but you are not sure you are ready to let go because it gives you pleasure or meets some need in your life (for example, food, drugs, alcohol), then that needs to be the first issue you work on. Many times when people don't heal as quickly as they expected, it's because of conscious conflict.

Continuing to do what you know is wrong when you know it is wrong falls into the "harmful actions" category in The Healing Codes system. (More on that in the next chapter.) It is one of the inhibitors of healing, and can be one of the most difficult areas to heal. However, change will occur as you heal the other issues that contribute to the problem. To remove the blocks to healing created by harmful actions and conscious conflicts, all you need to do is to desire to change, and then begin taking even the tiniest baby steps in that direction. As you continue to heal all the areas of your life, choosing only healthy actions will become easier and easier.

I notice other things are changing for the better even before my main issue goes away. Why?

Other things may change before the problem that bothers you most because they are related to your primary issue. The body will prioritize what needs to be healed in order to heal the source of the problem, not just the symptoms. If you don't allow this to happen then the problem often comes back. Most issues in a person's life are connected, so you are actually working on a number of issues at once. In order to heal the problem issue at its source, other things may have to heal as well.

After I do the Code, I seem to see things differently, even things that were not being worked on. Why?
Your body is automatically finding and healing the pictures and beliefs connected to your problem or issue. People often tell us they don't see things the way they used to before going through the process and doing The Healing Code. As their pictures have changed, so have the lenses through which they view the world.

Example: Remember the rape victim mentioned in Chapter Five? Asked what she felt about the rapist before doing Healing Codes, she replied, "I wanted to get a shotgun and blow his head off!" After doing Healing Codes for several days, something changed. She said that when she thought about her attacker, she felt pity and compassion for the man who raped her, and she was finally able to forgive him. Her pictures had changed and shortly thereafter her problems healed.

How can I tap into the positive experiences I have had in my life?
Try to focus on "love pictures" while you do your Code. Identify what we call a Love Picture by thinking of one or more individuals in your life who loves you. These can be people from the past or present, friends, family, even a much loved pet. We would encourage you to include God or Jesus on this list. Picture yourself surrounded and loved by those on your "love list"—what you are picturing is the truth. Picture them one at a time, or as a whole group. Relax and enjoy feeling their love touch your heart. If you are unable to find a Love

Picture, imagine being loved as you would wish to be loved. Caution: Some people have negative pictures of the people who should have loved them but didn't effectively express that love. Do not include these people; it can interfere with healing. Include only those whose love warms your heart.

Can The Healing Codes harm me in any way?

We quote again Dr. Paul Harris, internationally known lecturer and alternative health expert: "This is the only area of health where there has never in history been a validated case of harm." Of the many people who have worked with The Healing Codes, we are unaware of anyone who has ever been harmed.

Is this like…?

Even though The Healing Codes may seem similar to things you've heard of or done before, it is completely different. It isn't based on Chinese medicine, chakras, or acupuncture systems. The theory and exercises are unique to The Healing Codes system, although it clearly is working on the entire human energy system as well as everything else.

What if I don't remember any earlier picture?

You may not always know the picture you are working on, but your heart always knows. Your heart will automatically connect with each picture related to your issue. You will usually feel the healing of these pictures even though you may not be conscious of what they are.

What if I don't remember anything from a young age?

Sometimes individuals have blocks because of traumas. A trauma may be anything that unsettles an individual's heart, at any age. Sometimes a memory comes after doing several Code sessions. Since the Code works on an unconscious level, it is not necessary that you consciously remember the picture.

My parents never treated me badly. How can they be related to this issue?

It's great when you've had a good relationship with your parents. Sometimes, however, the unconscious doesn't always interpret events the same way our conscious mind does. So, to your adult self, a picture you remember may not seem to be a big deal even though it was a very big deal at age five. Remember the popsicle story!

How can this help my headaches (or other physical problem)?

With headaches as your issue, you will work on the image in your heart that is connected to the headaches. When the pictures are healed, stress will be removed from your body and your headaches will usually get better as your body functions as it was meant to. (Remember, The Healing Code does not work on headaches or any other physical issue— only destructive images.)

This doesn't work. My headaches are gone but I still have cancer.

Remember, we are only working on pictures. I'm glad your headaches are gone, and I hope your cancer is healed soon as well. But we are only working on pictures of the heart. We hope you can be thankful for the headaches being gone, and continue to remove stress from your body by doing the Code. This will free your body to use its energy on the cancer.

What if I only do the Codes two times per day instead of the three times you say is optimal? Will it still work?

Your Healing Code is always working. It just works more slowly if you spend less time on it.

What if I miss a day?

Try not to miss a day, as consistency is very important to the process. If you do miss a day, just continue the next day, and try to focus on doing the work daily. Healing will still occur.

What if The Healing Code stops working?

Our experience is that the Code is always working. There may be times when you don't feel changes happening, or changes are not happening as quickly as you want them to. Your feelings don't equal your healing. In fact, we have had many testimonials of healing weeks or months after the last time they did the Code.

WHAT IF HEALING DOESN'T HAPPEN?

If after taking all the suggestions above and doing your Healing Code faithfully three times a day or more, you don't experience any healing for your important issue, you may be wondering what's going on, is this for real?

The first place to look for an explanation is your own heart. You need to be honest with yourself and determine whether you are experiencing conscious conflict, as described above. It is the primary cause found to slow down healing. Conscious conflict can involve anything from dangerously harmful actions to eating poorly. It can also be something someone else is doing that you choose to remain a part of, such as putting up with abuse in a relationship. It slows down healing when you constantly create more destructive images and stress that need to be healed.

Is some element of your life in conflict with your own values? All of us have some conscious conflict. We have found that if you are taking even the tiniest steps toward living what you believe is right, it usually eliminates the conscious conflict that will otherwise slow down your healing. If you are not getting the results from The Healing Code that you would like, look for conscious conflict and let that be the first issue you work on with the Code.

The second place to look is how you practice the Code. Do you choose a quiet, peaceful time and place? Do you keep your mind focused on peaceful and positive thoughts or images, such as a positive Truth Focus Statement or a Love Picture? Do you do the full amount of time and number of repetitions, at the very least? Do you do the Code consistently every day?

We realize that most of our testimonials report rapid progress, sudden changes, and sometimes even miraculous results in both physical and emotional problems. Most of the people who take the time to write to us do so because they are excited and grateful at what has happened so quickly for them. Gradual progress inspires a lot fewer emails, but please note that we do have those testimonials, too.

Why doesn't everyone experience miraculous healing? It really makes more sense to ask why anyone *does* experience this healing. The Healing Code does not target physical problems. It doesn't even target emotional problems directly. The Healing Code targets only the healing of the heart issues outlined in the twelve spiritual issues addressed in the Heart Issues Finder (see next chapter, or go to www.thehealingcodebook.com). It is still amazing to us that as these spiritual issues are healed, so many physical and emotional problems are resolved as well.

The example of the two clients with migraine headaches is a perfect case of the differences in healing. One man's migraines were gone in a week; the other man's migraines hung on for a year. The difference was that the second man had many unconscious issues and wrong beliefs, all interrelated and connected to the migraines. The first man had only a few straightforward issues connected to the migraines. Physical problems are a *symptom of underlying spiritual issues*. They are not the true problems.

If you track how the amount of distress you feel about an issue or a memory is reduced as you do the Codes, then you know that healing is occurring. Many clients note subtle but profound changes in their attitudes toward other people and life in general. They have less rage in traffic; they aren't as upset by certain people or situations; they sleep more soundly. These changes can happen so gradually and feel so normal and natural (as indeed they are) that you may hardly remember how frazzled things used to seem. The absence of something negative doesn't always make an impression unless something else brings it to mind. Noting these subtle changes is encouraging when you need to see progress.

Again, you may want to register your book and download the Tracking Changes document so you can note changes. Even though your main issue may not be healing as quickly as you like, seeing some of these more subtle changes will encourage you that healing is occurring.

One client told us, "I've been using The Healing Codes for more than two years now. Not all my issues are healed yet, but I've had healing in just about every area of my life: physical, emotional, spiritual, relational, and in my career. Often when I do a Code, shortly afterward I completely forget what the issue was that bothered me, even if it was a 9 or 10! The healing is sometimes subtle, sometimes dramatic, but always profound."

Using The Healing Code should begin to heal the issues of your life, whether they are physical, relational, or related to success or performance. We hope that its simplicity and its power will show you that the healing system explained in this book is indeed a reality.

In the next chapter, we will introduce you to a tool that will help you pinpoint your heart issues, thus greatly enhancing your experience of The Healing Code.

CHAPTER ELEVEN

Using the Heart Issues Finder to Pinpoint Your Issues

As you know by now, many of the issues that are bothering you have their source in cellular memories and are below the level of conscious awareness. The Healing Code gets at those issues, but it does work faster if you can pinpoint at least some part of your current issue.

It took me sixteen years and a team of experts (Lorna Minewiser, PhD, and E. Thomas Costello, as well as computer programmers) to develop what I call the Heart Issues Finder. This tool is the only assessment of its kind that gets at these heart issues, which as you know by now are the source of all the problems you experience. My doctoral program had an emphasis on psychometrics and the construction of tests. Drawing on this knowledge, my team and I created the Heart Issues Finder to pinpoint the unconscious issues of the heart accurately. After you answer the questions online, you are instantly given a 10-15 page personalized report of your issues.

We have found that every problem a person can have in life falls into one (or more) of twelve categories. These are delineated below, and the Heart Issues Finder will give you results in each of these twelve categories. After we explain these categories, we'll show you how to use the Healing Code and the Heart Issues Finder to bring healing to any area of your life, from this point forward.

Here's an overview of the Twelve Categories which the Heart Issues Finder assesses.

Category #1: Unforgiveness

Category #2: Harmful Actions

Category #3: Wrong Beliefs

Category #4: Love vs. Selfishness

Category #5: Joy vs. Sadness/Depression

Category #6: Peace vs. Anxiety/Fear

Category #7: Patience vs. Anger/Frustration/ Impatience

Category #8: Kindness vs. Rejection/Harshness

Category #9: Goodness vs. Not Being Good Enough

Category #10: Trust vs. Control

Category #11: Humility vs. Unhealthy Pride/ Arrogance/Image Control

Category #12: Self-Control vs. Loss of Control

Let's look briefly at the Categories and why they are so critical to healing problems at their source.

THE THREE INHIBITORS

We call the first three categories of The Healing Codes system the Inhibitor Categories. We use the term "inhibitor" because they inhibit life, health, and prosperity. Because of this, for permanent, complete healing to occur, they must be eliminated. Eliminated is a big word, and maybe none of us ever gets there completely. That's okay. Ninety percent or so will do just fine.

CATEGORY #1: UNFORGIVENESS

For years I had been lecturing around the world that I'd never seen a serious health problem where there was not an unforgiveness issue. Years later, I met Dr. Ben, who had been lecturing all over the world and saying that he had never seen a cancer patient who did not have an unforgiveness issue!

Unforgiveness is the first category because it may very well be the most critical. In the Lord's Prayer, it is the only issue that Jesus addresses twice. In our experience, anyone who has an issue in any of the other eleven categories almost always has a related unforgiveness issue. Many times, however, these people will say that they do not have a forgiveness problem, or have already worked through it, dealt with it years ago in counseling, or let it go in some form or fashion.

Unforgiveness is often betrayed by some form of anger or irritation or not wanting to be around a certain person. No matter what you call it, it can kill you.

Many people who are aware of their unforgiveness don't want to release it because they feel like they would be releasing the perpetrator from their crime. These people grossly misunderstand forgiveness. Forgiveness is enlightened self-interest. It releases *me* from the perpetrator. As long as I refuse to forgive him, I am tied to him, and the longer the process continues, the closer I get to being dragged over the cliff with him. Oftentimes, the person I refuse to forgive is not suffering at all from my unforgiveness. He or she is not giving the matter a second thought. So it's impossible in this case for unforgiveness to be hurting anyone but me. The most loving thing I can do for my family, children, friends, or neighbors is often to forgive someone else and release that person from my judgment of their perceived wrongs.

Having said all this, many people do legitimately try to forgive for decades, but are unsuccessful. I guarantee you that the client of mine who was raped tried absolutely everything she knew to try to forgive her rapist. She consciously knew that her unforgiveness was killing her and ruining her life. She was dying, and the stench of death was absorbed by everyone and everything around her. In spite of her good intentions, three years later she was only getting worse and her unforgiveness had become a mountain of rage and fear. Less than ten days of addressing her unforgiveness issue with The Healing Codes cut the rope that bound her to the perpetrator and the rape.

CATEGORY #2: HARMFUL ACTIONS

Destructive behaviors may be the biggest category dealt with in the world of self-help, counseling, and therapy every single year. This includes weight issues, diet and exercise, and all addictions. Because behaviors are a result of heart issues (remember Secret #7: "When the Heart and the Head Conflict, the Heart Wins"), they are very useful "warning signals" for determining where we have issues that need to be healed.

An interesting thing about behaviors is that there are many that are neither right nor wrong. It's *why* something is done, not just *what* is being done, that can make it harmful. For example, as I'm writing this it's my birthday, and I have every intention of having a homemade chocolate milkshake with heavy whipping cream, Breyer's all natural vanilla ice cream, and the best chocolate I can find. I can't wait, and I can taste it right now just writing about it. So, is it a destructive behavior for me to have a milkshake on my birthday? Absolutely not. It's time to celebrate and let loose a little! In fact, it would probably be more stressful for me to stick to my diet on my birthday while all my cellular memories are recalling many years of cake and ice cream. The other side of that coin is if I'm having a chocolate milkshake for a destructive reason. Let's say I had a bad day at work, and I wanted to drown my sorrows in the decadent depths of a chocolate milkshake. Or maybe I have chocolate milkshakes every day even though I know that can be unhealthy to the point of taking me away from my family at far too young an age. Same behavior done one time for the right reasons, and other times for the wrong reasons. In other words, the same behavior can be healthy or destructive.

Now, of course there are a number of behaviors that are always wrong, such as rape, abuse of a child, or stealing. Even these behaviors are never the source of a person's problems, they are always a symptom of destructive cellular memories. So why address them? Why not just focus on the underlying memories? That's exactly what we're going to have you do in this category. Knowing that I'm doing destructive behaviors can be a warning light on my dashboard indicating there are cellular memories that need to be addressed and healed.

All destructive behaviors fall into one of two categories: self-protection or self-gratification. When Tracey was depressed for the first twelve years of our marriage, she did both. In fact, we were laughing about that today at my birthday lunch. Tracey would fix a pan of chocolate chip cookies (the best you've ever had in your life—everybody thinks so!), then she would lock herself in her bedroom and hide under the covers to eat them. The chocolate chip cookies are a good example of self-gratification behavior, while locking herself in her room would be self-protection. These are rather obvious examples. Many others are not quite so easy to identify. In fact, many behaviors that people believe are healthy are actually being motivated by unconscious, destructive cellular memories.

We call self-gratification and self-protection the two reaction styles of harmful actions. But what are they reactions to? Most people would think they are to their current circumstances—financial struggles, relationship friction, career frustration. While these can contribute to stress in our lives, they are not the primary cause. The destructive reaction is a response to a reactivated cellular memory that contains a lie about your life. In the case of Tracey and her depression, the lies were common ones that many people believe without realizing it: "I'm not good enough," "people will hurt me," "my life is hopeless," "everyone is better than me," "I can't trust anyone," "my only hope for sanity is to perfectly control my circumstances." Tracey concluded that the best she could do was to protect herself by hiding in her room while consoling herself with the chocolate chip cookies.

You may be one of the people who believe similar lies if you have some destructive behaviors, but don't despair. We believe you have the solution in your hands.

CATEGORY #3: WRONG BELIEFS

As we've already discussed, Dr. Bruce Lipton's research at Stanford University Medical School showed that what makes us sick 100 percent of the time is the stress that is caused by holding a wrong belief about ourselves, our lives, or other people. These beliefs cause us to be afraid when we should not be afraid, and stress and illness are simply fear that has become physical.

You could heal any problem in your life, for the rest of your life, very effectively using nothing but The Healing Code and addressing your wrong beliefs. These wrong beliefs are the tumors within our cellular memories that spread disease and illness throughout our lives. They are radio stations that are broadcasting propaganda about ourselves constantly into our ears. After years of hearing these lies with no way to change the channel, we start to believe them and act on them.

We always do what we believe. And everything that we do, we do because of something we believe. If your beliefs are right, your feelings, thoughts, and behaviors will be healthy. If you're doing, thinking, or feeling something that you don't want, it is always because of something you believe. If you change your beliefs, your thoughts, feelings, and actions will automatically change. Sounds easy … where's the rub? As we discussed in Secret #5, the beliefs that need to change the most are protected by your unconscious mind from being changed because they serve as a 911 alarm to help keep hurtful things from happening again. That's why people try for a lifetime to change their beliefs but few ever successfully do it. This kind of change is the essence of the popular term over the last thirty years, "breaking the cycle."

I recall one client who started The Healing Codes for a physical problem. She called me very excitedly shortly into the process and said, "Something has happened and I need to know if it's normal." When I asked her what the something was, she said, "My beliefs are changing." I asked her if this was a good or a bad thing to her, and she replied, "Neither one … it's wonderful." She went on to tell me all of the things that she had done, with limited results, to try to break these belief cycles in her life. She had focused only on a physical issue while doing The Healing Codes because she did not believe those beliefs could change. Without even consciously working on her beliefs, they healed through The Healing Codes in a very short period of time. We hear stories like this every week.

THE CORE HEALING SYSTEM

Category #4 is the start of what we call "The Core Healing System." As the three Inhibitor Categories were created to remove garbage from our lives, the nine Core Categories are designed to instill the seeds that will grow into life, health, and prosperity. A healthy home is not determined simply by an absence of garbage, dirt, or clutter. It is defined by the life that is inside. The joy that permeates. The peace that makes it truly a resting place. The kindness that makes everyone that comes through feel cared about and at home. In other words, a loving place that transforms the hearts of those who live there or visit.

Each of the Core Categories works on a virtue that needs to be instilled, a destructive opposite that needs to be transformed, and on negative emotions and wrong beliefs that indicate where the person is on the continuum between the virtue and whatever is blocking the virtue. In the Healing Codes Manual, we go into great detail about what those negative emotions and beliefs are. The Heart Issues Finder will help you identify these things as well.

There is also one body system included in each core category. There are, not coincidentally, nine major body systems. Every organ, every gland, every bone is inherent in one of these nine body systems. The Core Healing system has been a major "ah-ha" to most of our clients since the inception of The Healing Codes. It is a correlation of the physical and non-physical issues that tend to occur together. This means that if you have a negative emotion but cannot identify any related physical problem, you can go to the core category that contains that negative emotion and find the body systems and organs that will most likely be affected by that negative emotion. Conversely, if the only thing you know is that your chiropractor says you have a problem with your adrenal glands, you can go to the category for the adrenal glands and discover what wrong beliefs are most likely dictating your life in an unhealthy way.

In the more involved Healing Codes system, you can look up your symptoms in the back of the Manual and find the category the symptom falls under, and use the Codes for that category to heal the issue. Because the Codes target specific symptoms, they tend to be the most powerful Codes.[21]

I can't count how many people have written and called us to say that they never would have connected a particular physical symptom with a particular non-physical problem. They say that the understanding of how the problem developed was invaluable to their healing and peace of mind. Many of these same people have told us of confirmation from medical doctors, alternative therapists, and others that they did, indeed, have a physical problem in a certain area that had not manifested to the point that it was noticeable yet. The way the client found it was through the correlation of the Core Healing System. For instance, a client with low self-esteem learned from The Healing Codes that low self-esteem tends to

---

21 For more about The Healing Codes system, see p. 292 or visit
   www.thehealingcodesbook.com.

show up in glandular and hormonal problems. Even though the client didn't have any symptoms in that area, he went and had it checked out, knowing that the stress from low self-esteem had been operating on him for decades. The early detection of the physical glandular and hormonal problems his health-care provider discovered made the issues much easier to deal with than if they had not been addressed until they were noticeable.

CATEGORY #4: LOVE VS. SELFISHNESS

Love is the virtue from which all other virtues flow. The Beatles really did have it right: "All you need is love." Jesus was asked, "Is there one thing that is most important?" His response was, in essence, "Absolutely. Love." In fact, he went farther than their question and said, "If you love, you've done everything." If you have plenty of love, inside and out, everything else is usually okay. If you get love inside and out, anything and everything usually heals very quickly.

Before we go any farther, since love is the most important virtue, let's make sure we're on the same page about what love is. This is particularly important since the word is used for anything and everything, it seems. "I love chocolate," "I love these pants," "I love baseball," and on and on. Often, the word "love" is used in a way that actually describes the opposite of love, which is, of course, selfishness. Love, true love, is getting out of my own needs and desires to the point of doing what's best for other people and myself. If the choice is my own need or desire vesus the good of another person, love will choose the other person. This is one of the major things that separates us from animals who operate by instinct.

"Love" means choosing pain. If you've ever truly loved, then you have no doubt that love is pain. If I had divorced Tracey the first time I did not feel love for her, we would have divorced before we ever got out of the church. I must have heard, "One more picture," forty times, and my face was about to crack from smiling, and I was dying for a piece of cake. But love overrides pain and chooses to do the best thing in all circumstances. Does that mean that I don't ever get my needs met? Absolutely not. It would be very difficult, if not impossible, for me to love others without loving myself. The problem is that most of us are obsessed with ourselves or so in bondage to our destructive memories that we often don't even see the opportunities to show love to other people.

Love is also not sex. I say this because that may be the very biggest misconception in our society. Sex is not *making* love. Sex is supposed to be a celebration of love. I remember the old high school line used by many guys whose hormones were raging for sex, saying to an often gullible date, "If you really loved me, you would...." If he really loved her, he would never say that. While this example of teenage sex is amusingly obvious to most adults, we often operate under the same motivation with different behaviors. Addictions to television, the Internet, sports, or even good books can become love substitutes that obsess us and take us away from the intimate, loving relationships that we are built to enjoy.

On the other hand, a lack of love is the root of virtually every problem we can have. The body system for the Love Category is the glandular/hormonal or endocrine system. Just as every other virtue flows from love and every negative thing flows from selfishness, so the endocrine system is a vital part of every known disease or illness. Could you say that this is the most important category, even though we made that same statement about Unforgiveness? A strong point could be made for this, because unforgiveness is the result of selfishness or a lack of love. In fact, unforgiveness is one of the secondary components of the Love Category.

Doing The Healing Code on this category will heal love, selfishness, and endocrine problems. Even though we've said it several times before, it's important to say it again: The Healing Code doesn't address any physical illness or disease even though we just mentioned the endocrine system. The focus of the Code is always on the cellular memory, wrong belief, or negative feeling.

CATEGORY #5: JOY VS. SADNESS/DEPRESSION

Joy is often the easiest category to use to determine if someone is dealing with destructive heart issues or not. Joy is one of those things that is the most faked in modern life. Everyone wants people to think that they are doing well, so we "put on a happy face."

However, the presence or absence of true joy is a very good indicator of where the person is in their unconscious mind. Joy is one of the first things that goes when physical or non-physical problems manifest. Many people confuse true joy with happiness, but in our experience, happiness is based on our circumstances. If things go well, I feel good. If things go badly or don't meet my expectations, then I'm bummed (another technical term).

Joy, on the other hand, is a rare flower. It blooms in spite of circumstances. One of my favorite things is to be walking down the road and see the single flower that is blooming up through a crack in the hard concrete. I just want to stop right then and there and applaud and say, "You go, baby!" This is true joy. It is the indomitable spirit that we recognize in giants like Mother Teresa and Victor Frankl, who went through hell on earth and came out the other side not only intact, but better for it. True joy blooms in the soil of love. Where there is love, there is joy. An absence of love will correlate to a lack of joy every time.

The body system related to the Joy Category is the skin (integumentary system), which is the largest organ of the body. In my years of counseling and therapy, I rarely recall a depressed client who did not have some sort of skin issue. I know this was definitely true for Tracey, who regularly complained about skin problems and constantly picked at bumps on her arms while she was depressed. After teaming up with Dr. Ben, it was fascinating to me to hear him lecture that he had never encountered a depressed patient who did not have skin problems of some kind.

Sadness and depression are rooted in cellular memories whose lie is that life is hopeless because of something that has happened in the past.

CATEGORY #6: PEACE VS. ANXIETY/FEAR

Peace is the best indicator of heart health (the mind/conscience/spirit heart). Why? It is the only one of the nine Virtues that you cannot work to create more of through effort. It is the natural result of a loving heart. You can intentionally be more joyful, patient, trusting, self-controlled, or kind, whether that's where your heart is or not. Why would you do that? Because these things are socially acceptable in most cultures. While it's usually a good thing to cultivate these things, it still can be done from selfish motivation. Peace, on the other hand, cannot be developed in these ways. It is a consistent and predictable indicator of who you really are. You can choose to act in many different ways, but the presence or absence of peace is difficult, if not impossible, to manipulate for selfish reasons.

Peace is disturbed by fear, and fear is the parent of all negative feelings. Sadness, impatience, difficulty trusting others, counterproductive behaviors, self-indulgence, all originate from fear. Fear is a reaction to pain. Although all of us experience pain, some choose love and some give in to fear. The reason we choose what we choose is, of course, like everything else, embedded in the heart. Remember, when the head and heart conflict, the heart wins. Even if your conscious, rational choice is love, if your unconscious motivation is fear, the fear will win and will steal your peace.

I (Ben) remember seeing a bumper sticker that said, "If you have it, it was brought by a truck." If you have a negative emotion, it was brought by fear and, not coincidentally, if you have a physical ailment, it came through the Peace Category body system—the gastrointestinal system. The first time I (Alex) heard Ben lecture on the gastrointestinal system, I had so many "ah-ha" lights come on, I almost screamed. I never knew that just about every illness and disease originates in some way through the gastrointestinal system. Understanding that, it makes perfect sense that fear would cause problems in the GI system, since fear is also what causes all other negative emotions and beliefs. We hope you're seeing why so many people have been impacted so deeply just by understanding the correlations between their physical and non-physical health problems.

In order to avoid confusion, let us reference the Love Category, because we had said that every illness or disease known to man is related to the endocrine system. This is not in conflict with what we just said about the gastrointestinal system. They fit together with amazing harmony. The endocrine system is the first system in the body affected by our cellular memories and tends to impact the GI system first. From there, just about any problem you can name can develop based on your weakest physical link.

We don't want to leave this category without reinforcing one more time how amazing and critical this correlation is. Love is ultimately the source of all health, and the corresponding endocrine system is the first domino to health problems. If that first domino is never tipped over, it is difficult for any illness or disease to create a stronghold in your body. In the same way, selfishness, the opposite of love, is what causes us to choose fear over love. Once fear is chosen, negative feelings, thought patterns, and behaviors have an open door to derail the life we dream of.

We cannot emphasize strongly enough how important paying attention to your Peace/Anxiety warning light is to determine when you have a heart issue that's being reactivated. Even more than the Joy Category, true peace is resistant to circumstantial conditions.

How can this be used practically? For any issue you are dealing with, think about different variables, aspects, courses of action, and monitor your level of peace as you imagine the various possibilities. Often the best course of action will be the one where you experience the most peace.

Unfortunately, many people confuse true peace with giving in to fear. Let's say that for most of my life I've felt compelled to follow a particular career and a particular way of doing it, but for various reasons I've never stepped out and acted on it. My reasons could include finances, relationships, or maybe health issues. Now as I'm sitting down reading this book, I decide to test this course of action with my "Peace Indicator." When I think about actually doing what I've dreamed of doing all my life, I immediately feel afraid, and when I quit thinking about it, I feel better. This may lead me to confuse the relief I feel (from having my fear relieved because I changed the focus of my thoughts) with true peace. Very possibly the reason that I feel afraid when I think about doing the thing I've always dreamed of doing is that I have heart junk that is telling me, "It won't work for me," or "I'm not good enough, or "Other people can be successful, but not me."

This is how destructive cellular memories can dictate our lives, so it's important to understand the difference. What I need to do is work on that fear issue with The Healing Code and then test using the "Peace Indicator." The fear that I felt when I thought about living my dream is evidence that I have something to heal there. Lack of fear is not a part of the "Peace Indicator"; what you must feel is the presence of peace.

To elaborate, if using the "Peace Indicator" yields peace, that's easy—that usually means "go for it." If the indicator is saying "no," then what is usually experienced is not fear or anger or sadness, but something people usually describe as, "I just don't have peace about it." If you ask them, "Did you feel fear, anger, or sadness," their response will be, "No, I just didn't have peace about it." That's different from feeling strong negative emotions. When you experience strong negative emotions, it's almost always an indicator that there are heart issues that need to be healed regarding that issue.

CATEGORY #7: PATIENCE VS. ANGER/FRUSTRATION/IMPATIENCE

Patience may very well be one of the most underrated issues and categories. For some reason, we tend to put impatience in a totally different category from the other negative feelings and emotions.

However, impatience can be absolutely huge in a person's life. It is evidence that we are not satisfied. It is evidence that we are not content. It is almost always an indicator that we are comparing ourselves to other people, which always takes us down the wrong road. Comparing ourselves leads us to feelings of either inferiority or superiority. Either one is terrible and can lead not only to stress, but to every possible health issue. The tip-off for whether this is your issue or not is feelings of irritation, frustration, anger, or insecurity. Evidence of the pivotal nature of this category is found in its body system, which is the immune system.

The very first of the three "One Things" at the beginning of this book is that there is one thing on planet Earth that can heal just about any problem you have, and that is your immune and healing systems. We find that these immune and healing systems are most directly turned off by anger and its many affiliates, and by an unhealthy belief that "something has to change for me to be okay." Amazingly, when cellular memories concerning anger, comparison, and discontentment are resolved, physical illnesses tend to heal dramatically. This happens through turning the immune system back on.

The next time you feel impatient, correlate that with the fact that you may be, right at that moment, turning off your immune system and making yourself susceptible to illness and disease. A dear friend of mine who is here helping me right now just raised a wonderful question, and that is, "Wait a minute. I thought fear is what activates the fight or flight stress response that turns off the immune system." She is absolutely right. So, how can those two things go together?

Every negative feeling and emotion, including impatience and anger, originally comes from fear. Anger seems to be the indicator that the fear has gone far enough in someone's life to turn off the immune system. You cannot resolve the anger cellular memories without also addressing the fear. But you don't have to do that consciously. The Healing Code will do that automatically. When a person addresses his or her patience and anger issues, what we notice is that the immune system tends to turn back on in a more dramatic way than happens when addressing other issues.

This is also a good place to add that all of these correlations are merely tendencies, which we see exceptions to on a regular basis. You may never see a correlation between the physical and emotional issues in a particular category. No matter what your issues and correlations are, if you first work through each of the Twelve Categories, one per day, and then focus on the categories and issues that are the most bothersome (as indicated by the Heart Issues Finder), you will tend to heal consistently and predictably. In other words, there is something about The Healing Code mechanism that heals what needs to be healed without our having to have it all figured out. What a relief!

CATEGORY #8: KINDNESS VS. REJECTION/HARSHNESS

The Kindness Category may be the most critical one to the largest number of people, especially people who have experienced deep non-physical pain in their lives. A selfish person—one who is reacting in fear instead of choosing love—is likely to reject and be harsh with other people out of his or her own pain and feelings of rejection. This is the most devastating thing in life that anyone can experience—rejection from another person. It is at the root of just about any love problem (feeling accepted and loved and worthwhile) we can have.

It should come as no surprise, then, that the body system most affected by rejection is the central nervous system. While our cellular memories appear to be the control mechanism for healing every cell of the body (see Secret #3), the central nervous system would have to be considered the control mechanism for just about every other function. The millions of signals that coordinate the activities and movements of the body consciously and unconsciously are controlled by the central nervous system. Two of the most important parts of the body make up the core of the central nervous system: the brain and spinal cord. This drives home the gravity of rejection when we understand that the system most damaged by this rejection is the major control system of the body. Many people believe that as the nervous system goes, so the body goes. Therefore, the things most directly healing to the central nervous system are simple acts of kindness.

When I reflect on this, it's easy for me to see the remarkable truth in this association. The people throughout my life who have been the most kind to me are the same people I think of when I recall the people I love the most and who have loved me the most. Even though some of these people were only part of my life for a few minutes, they made a huge impact in my heart.

CATEGORY #9: GOODNESS VS. NOT BEING GOOD ENOUGH

A number of people have the Goodness Category as their primary troublesome category, especially people who have experienced emotional abuse, perfectionism, or legalistic religion. Guilt, shame, and fear are huge issues here. This has always been a big issue in my life, because I was raised in a loving home, but a rather legalistic religion. It took me decades to recover from my religious upbringing.

I can vividly remember a sermon by an old-time gospel preacher at a tent revival. I was twelve years old and the sermon was about hell, of the fire and brimstone variety. There was a particular point in the sermon when the preacher went on for a full three to four minutes banging his fists on the podium (which resonated because of its connection to the microphone), a scowl on his face as he repeated two words: "No hope. No hope. No hope. No hope. No hope." Every time his fist hit the podium and those words pierced my heart, I sank a little farther down in my seat. By the time the service was over and we left, I could literally hardly walk. I had a physical sensation that I don't think I've ever experienced again in my life. The only way I can describe it is that it was as if I had to go to the bathroom extremely badly, but I did not actually have to go to the bathroom. When we got in the car, I immediately buckled my seat belt and asked my dad to please drive carefully. This was back in the days when nobody buckled the seatbelt. In fact, my parents looked at me like I was nuts!

I was haunted by the fiery furnace image for days, until finally I could not stand it anymore and I asked Jesus into my heart out of fear. Believe it or not, this was a famous sermon that I would find years later on a record. I still have it today. For decades after that, any time I would do something that I considered sinful or wrong, I would have an enormous wave of guilt, fear, and shame wash over me. I did not connect it with the "No Hope" sermon. I simply felt like I was bad and did not measure up. This translated to my relationship with God, friends, teachers, and later, to girls. Guilt, fear, and shame can be absolutely devastating.

Besides the emotional distress, these feelings put our bodies in tremendous stress. A huge group of people whose issues are in this category are perfectionists. This is a tricky one, because a lot of people who struggle with perfectionism actually think it's a good, admirable quality, similar in some ways to being a workaholic. Workaholics are often praised for their hard work, so it can be difficult to see that it's really unhealthy.

Tracey's perfectionism has always demanded that she be perfect, or close to it, so that she will be loved. She received praise, warmth, and acceptance growing up when she did something just right, but she was oftentimes met with harsh criticism or punishment when she fell short—sometimes the tiniest bit short. So from then until now, Tracey has associated being loved with being "right." The obvious problem with this is that even the best of us can be wrong and mess up quite frequently. If Tracey's sense of worth is devastated every time she messes up, even if she got the twenty things before that one right, she is way out of balance. This was a significant part of Tracey's depression. After a couple of decades of trying to be perfect, she never could quite get there (though she was close). This finally turned into despair and hopelessness and, amazingly, the belief that she was bad. Why amazingly?

A few years ago Tracey and I told each other our biggest sins and transgressions. Whereas I rattled off my laundry list for hours, Tracey teared up as she told me most ashamedly about her biggest sin ever. When she was a little girl, she went with her dad to the hardware store, and as they were checking out, she saw those little tiny bags that they put nails in and immediately thought that one of those bags would be perfect to hold some of her Barbie doll accessories. She reached over (the little stinker), took one, and hid it under her coat. By the time she and her dad got to the car, she was absolutely wracked with guilt and sang like a jailbird to her father, after which she went back into the hardware store and gave the bag back.

That's it. That's the big, huge, gigantic, monstrous, "It's so bad, I'm not sure I can even tell you about it" of my wife's life. How in the world could a person so clean and innocent feel so bad and guilty and unlovable all her life? Because her heart said that's who she was. That was her heart programming. You see, the messages from our heart often do not even resemble the truth. Yet we still believe them, feel them, and act on them.

The body system for the Goodness Category is the respiratory system. When someone experiences fear, guilt, and shame, the most common physical reaction is difficulty breathing. I don't know how many clients I have had who, because they have lived in this category, told me at some time or another, "I can't breathe, I just can't get a deep breath, why can't I get a deep breath? Wait just a minute, I can't breathe." I had a client who was doing The Healing Codes and healing from breast cancer who has a remarkable testimonial in this regard. For years, she had not been able to get a deep breath although she is very much into health and nutrition. She had read books, tried special exercises, alternated diets ... everything that she could think of, because she knew that deep breathing is critical to your health and that shallow breathing, over time, can be dangerous. In spite of all of her attempts, there was no improvement. Sure enough, a few years after the breathing issues began, she was diagnosed with breast cancer.

This client started doing The Healing Codes and addressed what she knew was the biggest issue in her life, which was in the Goodness Category. She was working on that issue for the second time when she felt the issue heal completely. At the instant that she felt it heal, she spontaneously took a huge, long, deep breath. She did not even try to take a deep breath. Her body did it involuntarily. From that moment until now, she has been breathing deeply with no problem. When this occurred, she was so excited she was literally dancing around her house. Her husband happened to be out of the country, but she called him on his cell phone. When he picked up, she said, "Hi, listen to this!" and breathed deeply into the phone. No "Hi, how are you doing?" just full, deep breathing. He became excited, too, and said over and over, "Was that really you? Was that really you? How did you do that? That's incredible!" She publicly said on a radio show that she believes this was when her cancer started to heal.

CATEGORY #10: TRUST VS. CONTROL

I was told of a study that fascinated me. Some brilliant person decided to examine the lives of truly great world-changing people through the ages. Jesus, Gandhi, Mother Teresa,

Abraham Lincoln, and many others were analyzed to see if a common thread emerged. The author was trying to isolate what makes people great. What causes lives to be changed? What consistently results in breakthroughs? In other words, how can we be better?

One common thread did emerge. You guessed it, every one of these great people—world-changing people, people we would all like to measure up to—were people who had the ability or had made the continuous choice to trust. Most of them trusted God more than people, which gave them perspective on which people could be trusted.

When you think about it, it makes a lot of sense. You can't love without trusting. Without trust, we always have a selfish, protective barrier that inhibits love. When we let that barrier down, unbelievable things can happen. What is the barrier that makes us want to protect ourselves and not trust? If you say, "Oh, that again," you're right. It's fear.

Does that mean that these great people who all were trusting people never had bad things happen to them that made them want to protect themselves? Of course not. If you read about Jesus or Gandhi or Abraham Lincoln or Mother Teresa, you won't read very far before you discover tremendous criticism, persecution, slander, attack—in short, the things that cause most of us to close the doors to our hearts. Once we close those doors, we tend to adopt a way of living that is the very foundation of just about everything destructive: it's called "control." Whether in relationships, your health, or your career, extreme control usually leads to slow death.

Here's an example from the world of health. I had a client who was extremely controlling about her diet because she was sensitive to many foods, a condition which was intertwined with an illness she had struggled with for years. Although she wasn't ill anymore, the years of struggle and pain had left her with enormous fear of a relapse. Food was maybe the easiest thing that she could control in that regard, and she could do it under the socially acceptable behavior of dieting. I saw her one day after she'd been feeling bad for an extended period of time. After testing her with a technique I use to discover whether something would be positive or negative (a form of applied kinesiology), I advised her to eat a hamburger. You would have thought I had suggested that she rob a bank or kidnap a small child! She was absolutely horrified. You see, her pain from the illness was resonating such massive fear inside her that it was almost paralyzing. Her only way of coping with the paralyzing effect was to keep her life as controlled as it could possibly be. I literally didn't know if I would ever see her again, she was that angry at me for suggesting this, although I had been as loving and kind as I possibly could be, because I knew in advance that she would not receive that suggestion well.

The next day she called me and sounded like a giddy schoolgirl. She recounted her experience and remarked that literally, from the first bite of a hamburger, she had started feeling better. Now, does she need to have hamburgers every day, and am I saying that red meat is a good thing for your diet? No. But in that situation, for whatever reason, physical, non-physical, or both, she needed to have one hamburger. Sure enough, it broke through her wall of fear and she's been a different person ever since. By the way, she still eats very healthily, but now it's not out of fear, it's out of love for herself and truth. And she occasionally enjoys a hamburger or an ice cream cone with no ill effects.

One last example before we peel ourselves away from this issue. You may recall the story from Secret #4 regarding Tracey and me when we got married. We had done everything conceivable to be prepared and ideally matched for a wonderful, happy, largely stress-free marriage, and yet less than a year later both of us wanted a divorce. Maybe the predominant reason this happened is that we both had our "picture" of what we wanted the marriage to be and, largely unconsciously, exerted control over the other person to try to bring our picture into reality. But because Tracey's picture did not match mine and vice versa, our controlling ways led to anger, frustration, misunderstanding, and ultimately to distrust, rather than love and intimacy. I believe this category holds the secrets to why so few relationships deliver what we want. I heard a statistic recently that approximately 50 percent of people divorce and many who don't divorce live in apathy, unfaithfulness, or despair. At best, approximately five couples in a hundred experience the true loving intimacy that all of us seek and desire. The reason for this is rooted in the Trust/Control Category.

Knowing that, the body system that makes sense for this category is the reproductive system. Sex is supposed to be the height of loving intimacy. Loving intimacy runs on the fuel of trust. If you take away the trust, all you have is sex without the intimacy. Sadly, that's what most people have, and why so many people struggle with sex or look for a substitute. It's also very common in women who can't get pregnant or who struggle with reproductive issues to also struggle with trust and control issues. In fact, Tracey had three miscarriages and did not have a successful pregnancy for years. It was when she gave up control to God on a Sunday night in May that our first child was conceived.

CATEGORY #11: HUMILITY VS. IMAGE CONTROL

"Image is everything." At least, that's what a recent advertising campaign said. While down deep all of us know that's a lie, many of us still live our lives as if it were gospel truth. Image control originates from a belief that "I'm not okay, and if people get to know me, they will come to that same conclusion, so whatever the cost, I need people to see a manufactured me instead of who I really am." This becomes so critical to people who are stuck in it that they will often take any means necessary to portray a certain image or get people to think about them in the "right" way. We call this manipulation.

I will never forget going to church on Sunday morning with my parents arguing like cats and dogs. As soon as the car door opened and the first brother or sister said "Hi," my parents were miraculously transformed. They loved everybody and everything, and were madly in love with each other and their children. The world was a wonderful, fabulous place, and my dad's handshake with the preacher and hearty response of "Great!" left me disillusioned. I later found out that everybody does this. Somehow or another, it becomes built in that we need people to see us in a certain way. I think wanting to be liked starts way back before kindergarten for most of us and carries through our whole lives. That's okay—part of being human.

The problem comes when this causes us to put our energy into something that's not real—image. Of course, we want to put our energy in the place where it will pay dividends—

substance. We are who we really are in our hearts (see Secret #6). If we will put our energy into cleaning up our heart junk, we will automatically get what we really want, which is to feel good about ourselves. How other people feel about us will then take care of itself.

The circulatory system, which is at the heart (no pun intended) of our bodies, is the system most directly affected by these struggles. When we give in to manipulation and image control, we damage our heart, physical and non-physical. So to focus on my heart means to let go of many external things that entice me down the wrong path.

CATEGORY #12: SELF-CONTROL VS. OUT OF CONTROL

You may already be wondering if there is a conflict between the title of this category and our discussion of the evils of control a couple of categories back. The answer is "no." Here's why.

If we're not self-controlled, we can't love, we can't realize our dreams, and we will usually quickly destroy our health. So what's the difference? Self-control should not be a hard, forced, arduous task that is like trudging up a mountain in soaking-wet clothes. It should be more like skiing down a beautiful mountain on perfect snow. Self-control, when it is done right, is smooth and, at times, effortless. The difference is the condition of the heart. If our heart is in fear, then we will be trying to control to get what we need in order to be okay. If our heart is full of love and truth, on the other hand, we will be trying to control in love, joyfulness, and gratitude, because we're already okay.

Having said that, this has always been a big category for me. I am the youngest of three children and was spoiled within an inch of my life. My mother was the short-order cook, chauffeur, form-filler outer. In my senior year of college, I still didn't have a clue how to do laundry, balance a checkbook, or cook a thing.

This became a big issue in my life. I remember coming home from church on a Sunday morning shortly after Tracey and I were married, and while Tracey slaved away in the kitchen for an hour and a half, I plopped in front of the television to watch the NFL game of the week with a glass of sweet tea in one hand, a bag of chips in the other, and a remote in my lap. I can vividly remember becoming irritated with Tracey for making too much noise with the pots and pans, as I was having difficulty hearing John Madden and his play-by-play. After eating a lunch comprised of all my favorites, I quickly headed back to my recliner and became irritated again when the noise of cleanup interfered with the ballgame. My third irritation came about an hour later as Tracey had the audacity to disturb the exciting final moments of the game with her vacuuming. I'm ashamed of this now, but at the time, it was the way I was programmed. That laziness and sense of entitlement are critical issues in the Self-Control Category.

The muscular-skeletal system is the system most directly affected by Self-Control issues. It's been absolutely amazing to get reports from our clients reporting their muscular-skeletal problems healing as they heal the heart issues of laziness, entitlement, helplessness, fairness, etc.

PUTTING IT ALL TOGETHER

Now that you understand a bit of how the Healing Codes system addresses the physical and non-physical symptoms of heart issues, let us show you how to use this information to heal yourself both now and for the rest of your life.

Step One. First, we suggest that you start by using The Healing Code and working on whatever issue is bothering you the most. Go through the steps suggested on page 220: Identify the emotion behind the thing that's bothering you (fear, hopelessness, anger, anxiety, helplessness, etc.). Rate your issue (1-10). See if any memories come up of another time in your life when you had the same feelings, even if the situation is entirely different. Rate that memory in terms of how much it bothers you now. Include the memory or memories that surface, along with your current issue, in the prayer. Do the Code. When you're done, re-rate the memory. Keep working on that early or strongest memory until it's below a 1—you have perfect peace about it when you remember it. Then move on to work on any other memories that still have a "charge," starting with the next earliest or strongest, until they're all down to 0 or 1.

Step Two. Take the Heart Issues Finder. This assessment tool is online at www.thehealingcodebook.com (you'll get access to the link when you register your book). After you answer the questions, you will instantly receive a 10-15 page, personalized report of your score in the various Twelve Categories of Heart Issues.

This report will pinpoint the issues of your heart at the time you took the assessment. Start with the category of your lowest score. Look for any memories and feelings/beliefs that come up. Rate it 0-10, do the Code and work on it until the emotion is below 1 the same way as Step One. This may very well be the hidden source of the problem you worked on in Step One.

After you've worked on your lowest score from the Heart Issues Finder, work on the next lowest score (or the issue that bothers you the most, if something else has come up). Continue working with the Heart Issues Finder until you have addressed all your issues as the scores indicated. You can use this tool as many times as you like, and we recommend you do so. Not only will it enable you to know which issues need the most healing at any given time, it will also enable you to track your progress in the various categories.

Step Three. After you've brought up your lowest scores on the Heart Issues Finder, go through the Twelve Categories from this chapter, one per day. This ensures that you address all issues (remember, 90 percent of the source of your issues is unconscious). You can continue this "maintenance" schedule for the rest of your life. When a problem comes up, go back through Steps 1-3 and continue to heal the source of your issues.

FULL HEALING AHEAD

You now have in your hands the key to what we believe is the most powerful healing system discovered to date. You have the universal Healing Code that works for anyone, for any situation. You have access to the Heart Issues Finder, to guide you in assessing you heart issues and knowing how to prioritize the healing of them. You have the Twelve Categories, with which you can use The Healing Code to cover all the physical and non-physical sources of your issues.

Yet, guess what—we're not done with your healing!

The Healing Code and the Heart Issues Finder deal with the source of your stress on the cellular level. What about the everyday stresses, the kind of stress we usually think of when we think of stress? You know, when your child throws a temper tantrum, or you're stuck in traffic, or you've had an argument with someone.

We want to give you yet one more tool, this time to deal with the circumstantial stress of your life. In the next chapter, you will learn how to reverse these kinds of everyday stresses—in a matter of seconds!

CHAPTER TWELVE

Instant Impact:
The 10-Second Solution to
Situational Stress

No doubt you've seen the ads on television, the Internet, in stores—nearly everywhere you turn, drinks (and pills) are being touted for giving you an added boost in energy whenever you need it. It's a multi-billion dollar industry.

These concoctions are made up of certain vitamins and herbs that supposedly boost the effects of the caffeine they almost always contain. What they promise is hours of energy. But if you look closely at the ingredients, you see that it's another case of swapping a short-term solution (a temporary boost in energy) for long-term complications. Even vitamins and herbs can cause side effects when you take too much. Some energy drinks even issue a warning as to how many cans you can consume without harmful effects.

These drinks and pills actually add stress to the body by over-stimulating it and masking fatigue that is supposed to lead you to rest and relax, not get more hyped up. Most contain sugar, which suppresses the immune system, or sugar substitutes, which many believe are harmful.

What if you could get a similar or greater energy-boosting effect, without the stimulants, the cost, the "crash" you feel when the effects of the stimulant wear off, or the concern over side effects? What if you could tap this "energy booster" any time you wanted, without cost or inconvenience of buying anything, all in a matter of seconds?

And what if, in addition to the energy boost, you could decrease any negative emotions you feel and defuse stress—all in 10 seconds?

That's exactly what the Instant Impact exercise will do for you. Any time you are stressed, any time you need an energy boost, any time negative emotions threaten to overcome your peace of mind, "take 10." Take 10 seconds to deal with the stress—again, not by masking it with taking stimulants, which just add to your physiological stress level—but by *getting at the source and eliminating it.*

It is crucial to get at the source of your stress because of the devastating effects of stress on your body and mind. We've given you the tools to heal stress on the *cellular* level, the kind of stress that's usually activated unconsciously. But we all know there's another kind of stress that is all too conscious. Let's look again at this kind of stress, what it is and when and why it's harmful.

STRESS REVISITED

Stress is the natural and sometimes appropriate way your body reacts to a situation that causes fear or seems overwhelming. Stress is necessary for us to rise to meet the challenges of life.

Stress occurs when your mind believes that you are in some kind of danger—whether emotional or physical. It occurs when your mind believes that you don't have the ability to deal with an urgent situation. Your body pumps adrenaline into your system to give you a boost. This is called the "fight or flight" response.

Unfortunately for people in modern society, that adrenaline boost is physical, and it must be used by physical activity. If you do not burn it off by fleeing or fighting, the adrenaline remains in your body, creating tension and emotional distress. Too much stress without relief can leave us strained and drained, unable to meet daily demands with the balance and clear thinking that we need. We are tense, irritable and tired, and we can't figure out why.

Ideally, only life-threatening situations would trigger the stress response, enabling us to act quickly with less thought and faster reflexes. But today this response is often triggered by a ringing phone, a deadline, a boss, a family member, or any number of other non-life-threatening situations. We are continually bombarded with demands, expectations and unmet wants as we go through our daily lives. After being pumped full of adrenaline that we do not burn off, we are left exhausted, with a low-functioning immune system and a pervasive depletion of physical, emotional, and spiritual resources. This is when we might be tempted to reach for an energy drink. However, if we do, we're just masking the discomfort and adding more stimulation—stress—to our bodies.

Just as circumstances and lifestyles differ widely, so do the degrees to which people find events and situations to be stressful. What causes fear and overwhelm for your neighbor may not affect you the same way. Even so, all of us have our triggers and circumstances we can't face as well as we would like. This is called *situational stress*.

Some common causes of situational stress:

>Job-related issues
>
>Financial insecurity
>
>Fear of failure or of performing poorly
>
>Uncertainty about the future
>
>Health problems
>
>Family issues
>
>Relationship problems
>
>Dealing with negative people
>
>Holding negative attitudes
>
>Feeling powerless
>
>Low self-esteem
>
>Losing something or someone important

WHY GET STRESSED OVER TOO MUCH STRESS?

Because the long-term effects of continual stress are dangerous—even deadly—to our health and happiness.

As this very incomplete list of common causes of stress illustrates, situational stress is everywhere. It is so pervasive it affects our relationships, our work, and our ability to enjoy life to the fullest. High levels of stress leave us irritable and even angry with the people and circumstances around us. Family arguments and road rage are two common results. When we don't think clearly because of stress, we are inefficient and make more mistakes, which only increases our level of distress. In time, our stress levels build to a point where our immune systems are compromised and we are more prone to get sick.

When *situational stress* builds up over time, it creates a level of *physiological stress*. And it is physiological stress that causes almost all illness and disease, as you've already learned in Part One on The Seven Secrets. Stress shuts down important functions in our cells and, over time, our health suffers.

As we have seen, fight or flight is a necessary response to save our lives in emergencies, but this state of physical alarm should not be maintained beyond the time it is needed. The problem is that the average person is staying in fight or flight for long periods of time. When this happens, there is one inevitable result: eventually something breaks and shows up as a symptom. When we get a number of symptoms, we call this a disease.

UNRELIEVED STRESS IS THE ISSUE

Earlier we referred to the "stress barrel" theory coined by Doris Rapp, MD, who is considered by many people to be the premier allergist in the world. As long as our barrel is not full, we can have new stressors come into our lives or our bodies and deal with them quite effectively so they don't affect us negatively. Once our barrel overflows, our weakest physical area breaks down in some way. An allergy or a disease is simply where a weak area broke down under the pressure called stress.

In his book, *The Single Cause and Cure for Any Health Challenge*, Ray Gebauer, PhD, describes a dramatic study on the effects of unrelieved stress on mice:

> "When mice are placed on an electric grid and given very mild shocks, they are unaffected *as long as they are given enough time to recover from the stress of the shocks*. But if these mild shocks are too frequent, the mice are not able to

recover from this harmless stress, and they die from old age within a few short days. Even though each electric shock itself was harmless, *the accumulative effect of frequent stress* without enough recovery time *causes the body to just give up and die.*"

The implications of this study for people are pretty clear:

When we don't have enough time to recover from each stressful event before the next one comes, our cells stay shut down, our bodies age, and we can die before our time.

Some common effects of excessive situational stress:

> Insomnia
>
> Tension and anxiety
>
> Muddled thinking
>
> Inefficient action
>
> Increased errors
>
> Irritability
>
> Anger
>
> Mild depression
>
> High blood pressure
>
> Cardiovascular disease
>
> Heart disease
>
> Ulcers
>
> Allergies
>
> Asthma
>
> Migraine headaches
>
> Premature aging

We need a way to relieve this situational stress as it occurs throughout the day, simply, quickly, and without interfering with our already full schedules.

TOOLS FOR SITUATIONAL STRESS

Over the years, a number of effective tools have been developed to help people deal with situational stress. There are *physical approaches* such as vigorous aerobic exercise that promotes cardiovascular changes; deep breathing techniques; and energy medicine. All have been proven to release situational stress. The *non-physical* approaches to situational stress management, chiefly prayer and meditation, have also been proven effective. Probably 99 percent of the self-help material available focuses on either a physical or non-physical approach. Rarely is there any combination offered.

The simple exercise you're about to learn, however, combines *all* the proven elements of stress reduction—physical and non-physical—into one powerful exercise. We call it Instant Impact. And yes, it takes only 10 seconds to do!

Instant Impact combines, for the first time, the most stress-reducing physical and non-physical approaches known to date. In just 10 seconds you can feel as good as you'd feel after doing 30-60 minutes of vigorous exercise, deep breathing, or meditation.

Use Instant Impact any time you have an energy slump, or feel stressed throughout your day. It will interrupt the stress response so your body won't store up the stress but will get rid of it and keep you in balance.

For those of you who like to "get down to it," here's how to do Instant Impact. After that, we'll explain why such a short and simple technique is nevertheless so powerful.

HOW TO DO INSTANT IMPACT, STEP BY STEP

Instant Impact is designed to take only 10 seconds to do, though of course you can always do it longer. Most people feel results in the 10 seconds. We recommend you do it any time you need it, but at least three times a day.

Here are the steps.

1. Rate your stress. When you begin using Instant Impact, focus on the overall level of stress that you are feeling that day or that moment. How intense is it? How strong is it? How much is it affecting the way you feel? The way you relate to others? The way you see the world? Do you feel it anywhere in your body?

We ask you to rate your stress on a scale of 0 to 10, with 0 being no stress at all and 10 being an unbearable level of stress. This is an extremely helpful tool for you. When you rate your stress level before and after doing Instant Impact, you have a measurement for your success in reducing that level. You will know whether to do it again to lower your level further. You will know when your overall level of stress begins to decrease after practicing Instant Impact for a little while.

2. Place your palms together in any position that's comfortable. You can interlace your fingers, use a praying position, or any other position—as long as your palms are together.

3. Focus on the stress you want to leave your body— physical, emotional or spiritual.

4. Do Power Breathing for 10 seconds:

- Breathe rapid and powerful "belly breaths" in and out. Do this by forcefully blowing out and sucking in through your mouth. Use your diaphragm so your belly moves out as you breathe in and moves in as you breathe out. If you feel a little lightheaded, breathe the same way but reduce the intensity.

- As you do the Power Breathing, visualize something positive. It can be the stress leaving your body, or a peaceful scene, or whatever opposite thing you want instead of the stress. For instance, if you're feeling angry, you might envision or say in your mind, *patience*. Or *peace*. This is the "meditation" part of the exercise.

We suggest you practice this three times a day. Even if you do it once a day, you will see results. However, we highly recommend practicing this exercise three or even four or more times a day if you wish to quickly reduce your immediate stress and lower your overall levels. After all, it only takes a few seconds at a time—yet what a difference you'll feel!

You may be wondering how such a simple, quick, and easy exercise can remove stress and produce the effects of many more minutes of intense exercise or meditation. Here's how and why it works.

THE POWER OF BREATHING

Instant Impact uses a breathing technique called Power Breathing. *It is the Power Breathing of Instant Impact that allows you to interrupt the stress cycle and feel similar to how you'd feel after 20 minutes of combined vigorous exercise and meditation, in mere seconds.*

The physical Law of Inertia states that nothing changes unless it is acted on with enough energy, and Power Breathing creates tremendous internal physiological power. Power Breathing adds great force to this process—a high-energy fuel of oxygen and physical effort. Just as the wind is a primary source of power in the world, our breath is our personal source of wind power.

If you practiced only the Power Breathing, you would probably feel both invigorated and relaxed. Your mood would probably be lighter, too. It is an effective technique in and of itself, and it is the element that makes Instant Impact so quick and so deep.

Power Breathing addresses one of the effects of stress: shallow breathing. Habitual shallow breathing is a common sign of chronic stress. Shallow breathing begins with specific incidents that startle or alarm us, and it ends with becoming a habit. Chronic shallow breathing is like living in a state of constant apprehension.

In *Conscious Breathing*, Gay Hendricks, PhD, says, "When an emotion is very painful, our first reaction is to stop breathing. It's a protective fight-or-flight reflex triggered by the nervous system. Immediately after, you're flooded with adrenaline, and the sympathetic nervous system, which controls blood circulation, kicks in, making your heart beat faster and your breath quicken." Short, shallow breathing is the leftover of this response. Some people also habitually hold their breath when doing even small tasks. All shallow breathing reduces the amount of oxygen we take in and the carbon dioxide we expel, and this leads to stress at the cellular level.

Focusing on the breath several times a day will teach you to be more aware of your breathing. The belly breaths of Power Breathing show your body what it feels like to breathe fully and deeply. You will naturally breathe more deeply as you focus on letting go of stress or on feeling peace. When you continue to practice Instant Impact, you will begin to breathe more deeply between sessions. Your lungs will like the sensation of deep breathing, because it is more natural and healthy. Instant Impact should gradually increase your lung volume, a factor that promotes health and potentially increases life span.

As long ago as 1981, the journal *Science News* reported findings by the National Institute of Aging regarding lung function and longevity. A thirty-year clinical study of 5,200 individuals showed that a person's pulmonary function is a reliable indicator of general health and vigor and is also the primary measure of a person's potential life span. A measurement of pulmonary function can identify people who will die in 10, 20, or 30 years.

When you do Instant Impact, you will be more relaxed, and the muscles that control or inhibit your breathing will allow the full inhalations and exhalations your body is designed for.

Quite soon, you will find that you are more aware of when you are not breathing deeply. This will be a signal that you are feeling stress and need a break for Instant Impact.

With regular use, Instant Impact also:

>Stimulates the cardio-vascular system.

>Increases the intake of oxygen.

>Detoxifies the system of carbon dioxide.

>Stimulates the immune system by increasing energy to the endocrine system.

>Improves lymphatic system functioning.

MEDITATION

When you do Instant Impact, there is a simple "meditation" aspect as you focus on the stress leaving your body. Combining Power Breathing with Focused Intention—concentrating on your stress leaving your body—is part of the reason that Instant Impact holds for several hours. You are using the force of your breath to reinforce your intention and impress it on your mind and body.

Study after study has proved and continues to prove that meditation reduces stress and increases both physiological and psychological health. It is becoming an accepted medical fact that meditation enhances and increases a person's overall well-being. Although the process is not fully understood, research shows that meditation brings the brainwave pattern into an alpha state, which is a relaxed and peaceful level of consciousness that promotes healing. It also shows that blood levels of hormones and other biochemical compounds that show the presence of stress usually decrease with regular meditation practice. Across the U.S. and around the world, thousands and thousands of doctors, counselors and therapists recommend various meditation techniques to their clients as part of their healing and as a regular daily practice.

It can be surprising to learn that the medical profession—usually so very conservative—would recommend a practice that people think of as being spiritual. It's true that the primary definition of meditation is that it is a form of spiritual contemplation. Using a variety of techniques, people have used meditation for thousands of years as a vehicle for raising their level of spiritual awareness.

But meditation does not have to have a spiritual aim at all. The entire aim of meditation can simply be to shift your brain from stress mode to peace mode. Instant Impact incorporates meditation by inducing a very well documented "relaxation response" which stimulates particular areas of the brain.

A study led by Jon Kabat-Zinn, PhD, neuro-scientist at the University of Massachusetts Medical School, found that meditation shifts a person's brain activity from the right frontal cortex, which is more active when a person experiences stress, to the left frontal cortex, which is more active when a person is calm. This shift decreases the negative effects not only of stress, but also of mild depression and anxiety.

Studies by Dr. Adrian White at the University of Exeter produced similar results when he showed that people who meditate have increased electrical activity in the area of the frontal cortex, which indicates they are experiencing lower anxiety and a more positive emotional state. Meditation also reduces the amount of activity in the amygdala where the brain processes fear.

In other words, meditation literally moves our focus from fear and anxiety to peace. As you do Instant Impact and visualize your stress leaving your body, or a peaceful scene, you shift your brain waves from stress to peace.

ENERGY MEDICINE: USING THE HANDS

As you learned with The Healing Code, there is healing power in the hands. When you bring your palms together you are using the energy in your hands to defuse the stress. Again, it's a very simple yet powerful technique that enhances the overall stress reduction.

INSTANT IMPACT AND THE HEALING CODE WORK TOGETHER

There are stressful situations that are so complex and trigger so many negative emotions that doing Instant Impact only relieves stress very briefly. It takes The Healing Code to reach the cellular memories and wrong beliefs that are fueling the response to a situation like this.

Likewise, there are times when The Healing Code does not relieve the moment-by-moment stress of daily life. This conscious stress or even fear makes it harder for The Healing Code to work. It makes it harder for us to relax and let it work. It makes it harder to do it in the first place! When we clear away the circumstantial stress, when we clear away the resistance with Instant Impact, it seems to prepare the way to do The Healing Code. It's easier to do just about everything when using Instant Impact. In just 10 seconds, it removes a very high percentage of the resistance to healing.

The Healing Code works faster and better when we're not battling through circumstantial stress at the same time. In other words, The Healing Code does different and complementary things from Instant Impact. You need both to achieve optimal health.

We recommend you do The Healing Code three times a day, and "Take 10" with Instant Impact three times a day. That amounts to eighteen and a half minutes per day—a small investment with big results in your health, relationships, and success.

You now have the tools to deal with stress on the cellular and the circumstantial level. Wonderful as these are, useful as these are for eliminating stress at the source, we believe there are other components of a balanced, healthy life.

LIVING A BALANCED, BLESSED LIFE

Here are just a few more important suggestions in terms of living the most balanced, healthy (mind, body, and spirit) and fulfilling life—the kind of blessed life all of us long for.

Spirit. The first and most important component of a healthy life is developing a personal relationship with God. In fact, we believe that if you heal your life but do not develop a loving relationship with the Creator, you will never have what you need most—unconditional love. So we would encourage you to seek God and God's abundant love above everything else. The Healing Code can heal you physically and emotionally, it can help you become more successful in terms of this life. But it does nothing for your eternal destiny, and that is the most important of all. So we urge you not to neglect this step.[22]

Lifestyle. You need to develop a healthy lifestyle in addition to doing The Healing Code and Instant Impact. There are many commonsense ways to maintain your health and healing. These include eating nutritious foods, limiting unhealthy ones, drinking plenty of clean water, breathing clean air, taking vitamins and minerals, getting exercise and plenty of rest, spending time with people you love, and many, many others. You absolutely cannot live a balanced healthy life and neglect these factors, so please don't.

Under stress, both hydration and breathing are affected. Dehydration is the most common physical contributor to physiological stress, followed by insufficient oxygenation. Just drinking six to eight glasses of water a day and making sure to breathe deeply and completely can improve your memory

---

22 For more on what our personal spiritual beliefs, see "A Word about Us and Our Philosophy."

and energy levels, and decrease fatigue and general aches and pains. Their importance for health and healing can't be emphasized enough. The regular use of the Power Breathing in Instant Impact will improve the oxygen levels in your blood.

Conscious Conflict. As mentioned earlier, conscious conflict is when you are continually living something that you do not believe. It is the primary cause found to slow down healing because it creates constant stress. If you are not getting the results from Instant Impact or The Healing Code that you would like, check your heart honestly for conscious conflict. Deal with issues as soon as you become aware of them. Let that be the focus of your Healing Code work.

Self-talk. This is what we call "planting rotten seed." In his book, *You Can Love Your Life*, Dr. Neil Warren cites research showing that the average person has up to 1,300 words of self-talk per minute. These self-talk words are the brush strokes that paint pictures in our hearts. These thoughts are seeds we plant in our hearts that grow and produce.

If you are constantly planting new destructive pictures and beliefs while you are doing The Healing Code or Instant Impact, you are obviously "filling the barrel" and counteracting the healing effects. Consciously think about and focus on truth, love and respect for yourself and others, and anything else that is helpful and healing. Will you enjoy what you plant today, when it grows and produces? If not, start planting good seeds now! This is vital for long-term success.

OUR CHALLENGE AND OUR PLEA

In this book we have made some very bold promises.

We've said that a simple technique, which you can learn in 5 minutes and do in 6 minutes, can heal the source of any health, relational or success/performance issue you might have.

We have said that a 10-second breathing/meditation exercise can make you feel as good as if you'd exercised and/ or meditated for 20 minutes.

So we challenge you: Prove us wrong!

Go ahead and do these exercises regularly. For The Healing Code, a minimum of 6 minutes a day, two to three times a day. That's your prescription.

To deal with situational stress, do Instant Impact as needed, or three to four times a day.

If it really does not work for you, write to us! (If it does work for you, write to us as well. We'd love to hear your story.)

The only way these techniques don't work is if you don't do them at all.

Having said that, if you are doing the Code and feel stuck, or you want faster results, there is another level, The Healing Codes system, that tends to be more powerful because it's more specific to particular issues You can find out more about that on page 292. And when you register your book at www. thehealingcodebook.com, you can also get more information on the whole system.

But what you have now—The Healing Code, access to the Heart Issues Finder, and Instant Impact—will equip you to deal with the issues of the heart and circumstantial stress for the rest of your life.

Listen, if you heard about a pill that would heal whatever physical symptom you had ... improve your relationships ... knock out any blocks to success so that you can enjoy whatever success means to you ...

And if we said any time you needed this, for yourself or your family or friends, we would send it out, free of charge ...

Wouldn't you order a bottle right away? Wouldn't you order some for your friends and family and colleagues?

Well, we're sorry—this is not a pill! If it were, we'd probably have a billion-dollar product on our hands. (So people have told us.)

We apologize that we can't sell you a pill. Instead, we've sold you a book. Mere information. But information that you can draw upon for yourself, your family, your friends. Two simple techniques you've no doubt learned by now, that you can use to heal any issue of the heart, for the rest of your life.

Our challenge to you is to prove us wrong.

Our plea is to *use these tools* (even though they're not in pill form ☺).

And one more thing….

PASS IT ON!

For both of us, The Healing Codes is much more than a business. As the Blues Brothers once said, "We are on a mission from God!"

We want to see healing brought to the world. That's why we've written this book. Please, after you've read it and know how to do the Code, Instant Impact and where to access the Heart Issues Finder, loan this book to someone else who needs it. Teach the techniques to a friend over lunch. If The Healing Code and Instant Impact have helped you, tell others about it!

Help us spread healing to the world. God knows we all need it!

May God bless and guide you on your healing journey!

Going Deeper ...

A Word about Us and Our Philosophy

We've been to dozens and dozens of seminars, lectures and workshops over the years. We have read hundreds of books in graduate school, for training programs, and just for fun. We always appreciate it immensely when the presenters share what they believe, especially concerning their spirituality and worldviews.

We thought you might appreciate knowing that about us.

Simply put, we are followers of Jesus. We believe in one God, his son Jesus, his Holy Spirit who lives in us, and his written word, the Bible. We believe that God is the only being in the universe who is incapable of anything except love— because he *is* love. We believe that God knows and cares about each tear that falls from every person on earth.

I (Alex) grew up being taught that God was mean, vindictive, and selfish ... at least that's what I remember. It took me many years to get over my religious upbringing. I eventually came to realize that the Bible does not portray God the way my religious upbringing had taught. The Bible is a love letter. It does contain dos and don'ts, but so does the instruction book for my DVD player. The dos and don'ts are loving instructions by the Creator on how to live in love, joy, and peace.

We believe God calls individuals to certain tasks to spread his love. To us, what we are doing is not primarily a business, but a mission. We believe God has called us to the mission of helping hurting people through love. Some of this can be accomplished through the wonderful healing methods we sell.

Some of our mission can be accomplished by giving money generated by these products to programs with a mission similar to ours.

Currently, our main charity is a program in South America for street kids ages two through twelve. They take them off the street, give them a home, feed them, clothe them, teach them about God's love, and teach them a trade. In short, they give them back their lives.

So, in a nutshell, that's what we believe. If you would like to know more about our beliefs, feel free to contact us at www.thehealingcodebook.com. If you would like information on how you can help the street children, we will be happy to tell you.

Thank you and may God bless you!

Alexander Loyd and Ben Johnson

Register Your Book to Get Your Bonus Gifts*

Remember that when you register your book by going to www.thehealingcodebook.com, you will get several bonuses that will make this book even more valuable to you. You will need the book in hand to register.

Here is a summary of what you'll gain access to:

- Instant access to the **Heart Issues Finder**, the only assessment of its kind in the world that identifies your source issues and gives you a 10-15 page personalized report pinpointing the issues you can use The Healing Code to address. ($99 value)

- A video of the live event in which Dr. Alex Loyd and Dr. Ben Johnson revealed **"The Seven Secrets to Life, Health and Prosperity"** that a portion of this book is based on.

- Monthly editions of the **"The Secret Spiritual Laws of Nature"** newsletter from Dr. Alex Loyd sent via email for a full year.

- The **Personal Tracking form** you can use to keep a record of your healing journey.

- Sample **Truth Focus Statements** in the Twelve Categories to help you do The Healing Code.

- Invitations to teleseminars, news of research updates, and more. As new bonuses are added, you will be informed.

We hope you will "keep the dialog going" by registering your book, sending us your stories, and logging in to www.thehealingcodebook.com to keep up to date with all that's going on there.

---

*This offer is from www.thehealingcodebook.com. Hachette Book Group, Inc. is not affiliated with and does not endorse this advertisement/offer nor the www.thehealing codebook.com website, and is not responsible for the content of the foregoing.

More about The Healing Codes®

Now that you have The Healing Code and understand how and why it works, you may be curious about something we've been referring to throughout this book, the larger system behind The Healing Code.

As mentioned in Chapter Eleven, one of the key elements of The Healing Codes is the Twelve Categories. What you get in The Healing Codes package is a simple, easy program of exercises that address every possible problem and cellular memory issue in your life, whether you know you have a problem with it or not. After clearing many basic issues out of your heart with the "12 Days to a Changed Life," you can go to the Problem Reference Chart in the back of The Healing Codes Manual to find the problem that is bothering you the most. It refers you to the section of the Manual where you will find the right Healing Codes for that particular problem.

To learn more about The Healing Codes system, make sure you register your book at www.thehealingcodebook.com. You will then be able to access more information.*

If you are interested in hosting a workshop or lecture with Dr. Loyd, you will find information for that on the book registration site: thehealingcodebook.com.

---

*This is an offer from www.thehealingcodebook.com. Hachette Book Group, Inc. is not affiliated with and does not endorse this advertisement/offer nor the www.thehealing codebook.com website, and is not responsible for the content of the foregoing.

Index

About the Authors

Dr. Alexander Loyd is an ordained minister and worked for ten years in full-time ministry before earning doctorates in both naturopathic medicine and psychology. For a number of years, Dr. Loyd had a successful private practice in counseling and later in alternative therapies. For twelve years, Dr. Loyd traveled all over the globe in search of healing for his wife Tracey's clinical depression. Dr. Loyd's search led him to various techniques that could eliminate symptoms of depression and other illnesses, but not permanent, consistent healing. Dr. Loyd then poured himself into the study of energy and quantum physics.

In the spring of 2001, Dr. Loyd discovered a simple, physical mechanism that eliminates stress in the body by healing its source, which to his amazement and delight, healed Tracey's depression quickly. For the next year and a half Dr. Loyd validated this mechanism through Heart Rate Variability tests: the state-of-the-art mainstream medical diagnostic test for measuring stress in the autonomic nervous system. In 86 percent of cases, stress was virtually eliminated from the body within 20 minutes. Previous to Dr. Loyd's research, six weeks was the least amount of time any modality had been documented to consistently balance the autonomic nervous system, according to available literature going back thirty years.

Based on his discovery, Dr. Loyd founded The Healing Codes®, a company dedicated to natural healing around the world. To date, thousands of clients in 50 states and 90 countries have reported healing from illness and disease by activating the body's stress release mechanism with The Healing Codes. The procedure is non-invasive, there is nothing to take, and it does not involve diet or exercise. Dr. Loyd has trained 200+ coaches who work with clients over the phone, guiding them through this simple, natural procedure.

Dr. Loyd lives with his wife, Hope Tracey, and his two sons, Harry and George, in Tennessee.

Dr. Ben Johnson resides in Georgia, with his wife and seven children. He is a complementary and alternative medicine physician. He was clinical director of the Immune Recovery Clinic in Atlanta, Georgia, for several years, resigning in October 2004 to work full time with The Healing Codes after The Healing Codes healed him of his Lou Gehrig's disease. Never before had he experienced a therapy which allowed the autonomic nervous system to normalize in a matter of minutes, allowing the body to begin the healing process it was designed to perform. He now lectures around the world about The Healing Codes and how they work, and was the only MD featured on the popular DVD, *The Secret*.

Dr. Johnson served in the armed forces during Vietnam and was a flight surgeon in the Army reserve for many years. He was a Senior Aviation Medical Examiner for the FAA for twelve years. His major area of interest is cancer, and he devotes most of his time to researching and designing protocols for cancer patients. Dr. Johnson earned his first medical degree as a DO from University of Health Science, Kansas City, Missouri; his MD from The University of Science, Arts and Technology, Montserrat, West Indies, and his NMD from The United States School of Naturopathy in Washington, DC.

He is the Chief Executive Officer of Biopharmika, Inc. In his spare time, Dr. Johnson is a helicopter and a fixed wing pilot.